THE HOSPICE WAY

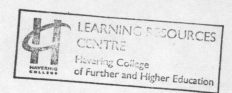

THE
HOSPICE
WAY

DENISE WINN

An OPTIMA book

© Denise Winn 1987

First published in 1987 by
Macdonald Optima, a division of
Macdonald & Co. (Publishers) Ltd

A BPCC PLC company

BRITISH LIBRARY CATALOGUING IN PUBLICATION DATA

Winn, Denise
    The hospice way.
    1. Hospices (Terminal care)
    I. Title
    362.1'75   R726.8

    ISBN 0-356-12741-9

Macdonald & Co. (Publishers) Ltd
3rd Floor
Greater London House
Hampstead Road
London NW1 7QX

Typeset by Leaper & Gard Ltd, Bristol, England
Printed in and bound in Great Britain by
Hazell Watson & Viney Ltd
Member of the BPCC group
Aylesbury, Bucks

In memory of my mother, Lucie

THE HOSPICE WAY

CONTENTS

INTRODUCTION

It is only in comparatively recent years that we have
become particularly concerned with the care that is
offered to people who are dying — and especially to those
dying from cancer, the disease which still causes most
fear. Once it was the norm for people to die at home,
surrounded by their families. Now, as a result of social
and economic changes, whole families are less likely to
stay together in one place, and women are as likely as men
to go out to work. As a result there may be no one at home
to care for a dying relative, and very many older people
end up living alone.

Medical advances of recent years, particularly
breakthroughs in high technology medicine, have focused
attention on cure rather than on palliative care. But there
simply isn't a cure for everything. One in five people die of
cancer, a disease that takes many forms. Some cancers do
not yet respond well to any known treatment, others

become fatal because they spread.

Despite the fact that the needs of people who are dying are different from those for whom treatment is possible, most people who die of cancer die in general hospitals. Just under a third of cancer patients live out the last of their lives at home, and only ten per cent do so in hospices or other specialist in-patient units designed to care for the terminally ill.

Although attitudes towards death are starting to change, and many doctors and nurses in general hospitals want to offer better care for dying patients, hospitals are essentially geared towards cure and treatment, not comfort and palliative care. Doctors are only human beings, and many are personally uncomfortable with death, seeing the dying patient as evidence of their own failure. In National Health Service hospitals, all staff are overstretched and overworked. They do not have the time, even when they do have the skill, to offer real comfort and understanding to dying people and their relatives.

Young nurses are often very upset by their first encounter with death. Though aware that someone is dying, the demands of their routine work and the needs of other patients may make it impossible for them just to sit quietly by and hold the dying patient's hand. Although most cancer patients die in hospital, many do so alone.

Doctors cannot be with patients all the time, and they often find it easier to cope by distancing themselves emotionally. In some hospital wards it is "policy" not to tell patients that they are dying, even when asked, because it is believed that the truth will only cause unnecessary misery and depression. Yet the result is very often that the dying person feels isolated and frightened.

Patients may realise something is very wrong because doctors cease to spend much time at their bedside during ward rounds, and questions receive only evasive answers. They may feel in awe of the consultant and thus express their anxieties only to the nurses, whom they feel they know better. But the nurses, if prevented by the "rules" from being honest with the patient, can only respond with cautious evasions or hearty untruths. This is an unpleasant and uncomfortable situation for them to be forced into, and causes more tension in the atmosphere for the patient to sense and worry over.

Relatives, too, may feel themselves excluded from caring for the patient. Less than generous visiting hours may restrict their time together; they may feel frustrated that they cannot help in simple practical ways because all the patient's physical needs have become the province of the professional staff. Although bound by no policy that prevents them from being honest with their loved one, they may themselves genuinely not know the severity of the condition, as doctors, in their own embarrassment, sometimes use medical terms which are not readily understood. And if it is hard for staff, who are not emotionally involved with the dying person, to face telling the patient the truth, it is even more frightening for the relatives, especially when there is no support they can count on.

It has been estimated that a fifth of the cancer patients who die in hospital suffer pain for which relief would have been possible, had communication been freer and had the staff known more about the requirements for symptom control in terminal illness.

Families who care for a relative at home do not, unfortunately, automatically escape these kinds of problems. A recent survey of general practitioners in north-west London showed that a third usually or always experienced difficulty in controlling a patient's pain; and nearly half had extreme difficulty coping with the emotional distress of relatives and patients. Without expert help and support, the tension and emotional pain experienced at home may be as great as in the hospital ward.

My sister and I experienced the emotional trauma of not knowing how or if to tell my mother that she was dying from cancer when we were caring for her at home a few years ago. In the end we did not, although we had so much wanted to be honest with her and share openly all that was happening. We worry still that we didn't do our best by her, despite our intentions. We would so much have welcomed skilled support and advice.

Twenty-eight per cent of people who die of cancer at home die in pain which could have been relieved. For bereaved relatives, no matter where it was that their loved one died, the terrible memory of their suffering is very often still strongly with them years after their death.

There is, therefore, a tremendously important place for specialist terminal care, which is what the hospice movement offers. Hospices aim to create an atmosphere of openness and trust, where emotional and spiritual pain can be honestly faced and relieved, along with the physical pain. They treat the dying with dignity, and respond to needs as patients themselves perceive them. They include and support the relatives, seeing this not as a privilege for the relatives, but as their right.

The hospice movement is still comparatively new, but already its specialist skills have become recognised by medical and nursing staff working in general hospitals and by general practitioners in the community. An increasing number of doctors are now trying to incorporate the hospice philosophy of care into their own work with the dying.

For hospice care need not be confined to a hospice. It is essentially an attitude and skill which, once learned, can be offered anywhere. Hospice skills are increasingly finding their way into the community — where support teams help families care for relatives at home; and into hospitals — where special wards or specialist teams can help meet the physical and emotional needs of the dying.

This book is about the special quality of hospice-style care, wherever it is provided. It aims to explain in simple terms exactly what hospice care means, how it works, and what it aims to achieve. Of necessity, I have talked about the hospice movement as if all hospices were the same. In fact they are not all the same. A vast number have been funded by money raised in the community and thus operate as independent units. They do not have to conform to exact standards in the way that National

Health Service hospices do. While this has advantages, in that such hospices are not part of any bumbling bureaucratic structure, it also means variation in the way that they work and what they achieve in practice. The common factor, however, is a philosophy of care. It is that philosophy which I have tried to describe here, in terms of how we, as caring relatives or caring professionals, can benefit from it in our care of the dying.

My thanks go to all the hospice staff who gave their time to talk to me; to the Hospice Information Service for the use of their extensive library; and to all those professionals who have shared their expertise in published papers, from which I have derived much insight as well as a very healthy respect for their superhuman caring.

1.

WHAT ARE HOSPICES?

COMMON MISCONCEPTIONS

The word "hospice" has become quite familiar in recent years. Most people, even if they have not had cause to know one for themselves, probably have an image of them as specially built homes dedicated to the care of the dying. They are places, some think, that people go into and never come out of again. They are therefore, perhaps, to be feared.

Neither of these images is accurate. Hospices are certainly dedicated to the care of those for whom cure is no longer a likely possibility; but they are just as much about living as dying. Many are indeed purpose-built, but hospice-type care can now also be provided within some hospitals and, increasingly, within a patient's own home. For a hospice is not so much a place as a concept in care which can, given the right support, be translated into many other settings.

~~

THE AIMS OF A HOSPICE

Hospices have three main aims, all of which stem from one vital principle: that a person for whom there seems no hope of cure is still a living human being, with hopes, fears and needs, and still with the capacity for giving and sharing; a person with the right to dignity and feelings.

The first task of hospice care is therefore to relieve pain and any other distressing symptoms which cause discomfort and fear, and debilitate not only the body but also the spirit. Only when someone is free of pain can he or she be free to live as fully as possible for all the time that is remaining.

But pain is not all physical. Much of what feels like physical pain can in fact be caused by anxiety about death, by fears for what will happen to loved ones, by unresolved emotional conflicts from the past, or by regrets for what now may not be achieved in the future. The second aim of hospice care is to create an open and safe atmosphere in which patients can gradually become relaxed enough to express fears and emotional pain, some of which may even be hidden from themselves, in the secure knowledge that their feelings will be treated with respect and gentleness, and that they will never be left to struggle with them alone. Nothing that patients don't want to hear is ever forced upon them; but neither are they fobbed off with dishonest or evasive answers when asking or hinting for the truth.

Thirdly, and just as importantly, in a hospice the emotional needs of relatives are also cared for. Whole families, including pets, are positively welcomed and seen as very important contributors (in some ways, the *most* important contributors) to the patient's well-being. Staff will work with relatives to help them uncover and face their own fears about death, many of which may be unfounded, and to ease the way for relatives and patients to be as open and honest with each other as they can, so that both can make the most of their remaining time together. Nor are the relatives forgotten after the loved one's death. Hospice staff are there to comfort and encourage the full expression of grief.

ACCEPTING DEATH

Some people feel uneasy about the hospice approach, seeing it as negative because it strives towards acceptance of and preparation for death, rather than towards every possible method of curative treatment, however slim or even hopeless. That is not how hospices view themselves. As Dame Cicely Saunders, the founder of the modern hospice movement, has said: "Accepting death's coming is the very opposite of doing nothing." For it is only after the acceptance of the inevitability of death, not necessarily today, this week or even this month, but soon, that someone who has limited hopes of life may let go enough to live it.

In many ways, the hospice has a great deal more to offer, and to elicit from, the patient than the hospital where, finally, the consultant reluctantly confesses, "There is nothing more I can do". True, there may be nothing more he can offer by way of hope of cure or temporary respite; but there is always plenty more that can be done for the physical, emotional and spiritual comfort of the patient. That is what hospices make time for. Their skills in symptom control, open communication and responding to individual needs are such that patients very commonly regain an unanticipated degree of independence and ability for self-care, as well as a new alert interest in life itself, however short. Hospice care, as one worker put it, is about active acceptance, not passive resignation.

But there is nothing didactic about the hospice approach to death. Staff aim to respond to needs as the *patients* themselves see them. The elderly dying woman isn't obliged to discover God or even to mention or acknowledge death if she doesn't want to. But she will be offered all the support and comfort she does want, whether physical, emotional, social and/or spiritual, and so will her family. People always come before routine, so a nurse will sit on the bed of a young man who wants to talk and just listen for however long he needs her and never mind the fact that he hasn't yet been shaved or had his shower.

The aim of helping people really live until they die is not a glossy euphemism for easing the passage to death. If patients come to them in time, hospices will help them live out their lives as they themselves want to, encouraging them to see that they can still give, achieve and enjoy a great deal within their own individual capabilities. That may mean being taken for walks in the park, at a time when a person was expecting never to be able to leave bed again; it may mean visiting the theatre; it may mean returning home for a visit or even to live. For someone else, it may mean overcoming a sense of worthlessness and withdrawal from life, and seeing that they can still play an important part in family decision-making; or repairing an old rift with a friend or family member; or simply achieving peace of a mental or spiritual kind. The priorities, whatever they are, are invariably the person's own.

THE FIRST HOSPICES

Hospices are not a new concept, although it is true that they have taken on a new form in the last couple of decades, a form identified by the term "the modern hospice movement".

In olden times, however, hospices were run by various religious orders, and were places where pilgrims and other travellers could stop and rest for the night and be given food. The name hospice came from *hospes*, the Latin word for guest. Gradually they began also to open their doors to the sick and dying who had nowhere else to go. The word hospice then became associated with care of this kind.

The most direct antecedent of the modern hospice movement was the hospice established in Dublin by the Irish Sisters of Charity in the late nineteenth century. In 1900, five of the Sisters came to the East End of London to carry on their work with the dying and, a few years later, set up St Joseph's Hospice there. By then, there were two other homes for the dying in London, one run by Anglicans and one by Methodists. But it was while working at St Joseph's that, some 60 years later, a young doctor named Cicely Saunders took the step that put the modern hospice movement on the map.

CICELY SAUNDERS

Cicely Saunders had trained as a nurse, but had to give up the work because of an injury to her back. She then became a medical social worker, and it was in St Thomas's Hospital in London, in the first ward she took over as a social worker, that she met the man who was to open her eyes to the inadequacy of care for the dying. His name was David Tasma. He was a refugee from Poland,

23

40 years old, and dying of incurable cancer.

Cicely became very close to him, since he had no relatives or friends, and they talked many times about how hospitals could provide much more loving care than they did for dying patients. Although the hospital did its best, David suffered much pain and discomfort, both physical and mental. It was then that Cicely first mooted the idea of building a special hospital herself, to cater specifically for the very different needs of the terminally ill. David was thrilled to be the inspiration of such an idea, and when he died he left her all his money (£500), saying "I'll be a window in your home".

After David's death, Cicely became a volunteer nurse at St Luke's, the home for the dying in London which was run by the Methodists. There she learned the nuns' practice of giving painkillers *before* pain reasserted itself, something not done in hospitals then, and rarely now. It was while at St Luke's that a doctor told her that, if she really wanted to help the dying, it was doctors' attitudes she must change, and to do that she had best become a doctor herself. So it was that by 1958 she had qualified, and won herself a research scholarship at St Mary's Hospital in Paddington to study the treatment of pain in the terminally ill.

Then she began work at St Joseph's Hospice in London's East End, and introduced there the pain relief system used by the nuns at St Luke's. In 1959 she began the mammoth task of planning her own special home, undaunted by the seemingly impossible task of raising half a million pounds to build and staff it. She badgered all and sundry for funds, and worked with an architect to design exactly the building she had in mind to fit dying patients' needs. She wanted to create a centre that could provide the best in nursing and medical care, as well as facilities for training and research, and where spiritual needs could be met but without any overtly religious overtones.

In 1969 Her Royal Highness Princess Alexandra opened the new hospice, called St Christopher's, in South London.

Though funded by grants and donations, its running costs are now partly met by the National Health Service and, to patients, its care is free. It has 62 beds and takes patients of any or no religion.

A beautiful yet homely building, with a wealth of windows overlooking peaceful colourful gardens as well as a road that hums with life, St Christopher's is still the inspiration and model for the modern hospice movement. It is a remarkable testimony to a remarkable woman, now Dame Cicely Saunders. And, by the large sunny window in its reception, is a plaque for David Tasma.

The fruits of the hard work of Dame Cicely and her devoted staff soon inspired others to try and raise money to build similar homes in other parts of the country. Hospices caught public and professional imagination because they returned dignity to dying, and placed value once again on the qualities of human caring, at a time when medicine had become increasingly technological and cure-oriented. They came, too, at a time when infectious diseases had ceased to be the main cause of death, and had been replaced by a growing incidence of cancer.

~

HOSPICES TODAY

Today there are nearly 100 in-patient units (providing in all over 2,000 beds) offering care for the dying broadly along hospice lines. Over half were built with independently raised funds, although a number have their running costs met, at least in part, by the National Health Service.

Established charities such as the Marie Curie Memorial Foundation and the Sue Ryder Foundation also have several units specifically for the care of the terminally ill.

Recent years have seen the establishment, by the National Society for Cancer Relief, of Macmillan

continuing care units (named after the NSCR's founder
Douglas Macmillan) on the grounds of National Health
Service hospitals, with running costs taken over by the
health authority. More recent still is a growing trend to set
up continuing care wards within National Health Service
hospitals themselves.

~~

HOME CARE SERVICES

Hospices with in-patient units increasingly see their role
as providing short-term symptom relief and a respite from
care for overstrained relatives. Another encouraging
development, the provision of hospice-style services in the
home, means that hospices no longer expect to be the last
resting place for all patients who come to them. There
are now over 100 home care teams in Britain and Eire.

About half of all hospices have their own home care
teams, but there are also a large number based in the
community. Most of these are initiated and funded, for
the first three years, by the National Society for Cancer
Relief, and are called Macmillan Services. There are over
300 Macmillan nurses countrywide who, with their special
on-call skills in the care of the terminally ill, have helped
innumerable families to care for their relatives at home.

~~

HOSPITAL SUPPORT UNITS

The last important development which is helping to
spread hospice-type care to even more people in need is
the hospital support, or symptom control, unit. These
have been set up in some district hospitals and are staffed

by specialists to advise hospital staff on the needs and care of patients dying in hospitals. Some also carry on a liaison role if a patient returns home.

What all these different styles of caring have in common are an emphasis on human needs, personal skill, one-to-one attention, and the availability of expert 24-hour on-call help — a combination that, with the right trained and caring staff, can be provided anywhere.

2.

WHOM CAN HOSPICES HELP?

Hospices, then, are very clearly not static institutions but a whole concept in care that, increasingly, is reaching out into the general community. It is simply no longer true that patients who go into the in-patient units are unlikely to leave again.

~

SYMPTOM CONTROL

Very many people go into hospices because their symptoms have become difficult to control in hospital or at home.

A large proportion are suffering severe pain which hospices are skilled at alleviating very quickly, but many have other physical problems which cause them discomfort, such as loss of appetite and weight loss, difficulty in breathing or swallowing, insomnia, nausea, bleeding or bedsores.

All these kinds of symptoms can be brought under control, and patients may then be discharged home again, in the knowledge that they can return any time they need to.

~

SHORT STAYS FOR OTHER REASONS

Over half of hospice patients are also likely to have social reasons for seeking admission. Some may be living alone, others may have families for whom the strain of caring for a sick relative has become, at least temporarily, too great a burden. For yet others, of course, their families, however caring, may be unable to look after them full-time because of their own work commitments.

It is difficult to give a meaningful figure to indicate the proportion of people who are nowadays discharged from hospices to live out their lives at home. There will always be those who, being elderly and lonely and having no one to care for them at home, will more happily remain in a hospice till they die.

Others may be brought to the hospice only at the very end of their lives, if their symptoms suddenly need expert control, and die within 48 hours.

LENGTH OF STAY

Experts believe it is best if people do not stay longer than
six months in a hospice. Despite the very warm and caring
atmosphere, it is sad and difficult for a patient to make
relationships with a great number of other people who will
inevitably die first.

Equally it is not ideal, from the hospices' point of view,
if people with whom they have had no prior contact are
with them for only 36-48 hours. This does not allow
enough time for the staff to give the psychological support
they are skilled at offering to either the patient or their
family. From that point of view, a stay of two to three
weeks is perhaps ideal.

NON-CANCER PATIENTS

Most hospices specialise in caring for people who are
suffering from cancer. There is no particular reason why
this should be so, except that hospices have become very
expert at caring for the particular needs of cancer
patients, and resources at the present time are too small
and too uncertain to justify spreading their net too much
further.

Cancer is still the disease which is most feared by the
public at large; at the same time, it is very amenable to
good symptom control by those who know how. And since
one in five of all deaths is from cancer, there are not
enough hospices to cater even for all cancer sufferers who
could benefit from their care.

The hope is that experts in other degenerative diseases
will perhaps, in time, take what they can from the hospice
model of care, and apply and adapt it for their own
patients. Certainly hospice-type care may become very

important for AIDS patients.

At present, however, only about one-third of hospices will accept one or two patients suffering from long-term diseases other than cancer. Most such patients are suffering from motor neurone disease, a progressive illness that weakens the muscles and eventually causes paralysis. The nursing care needed is more intense but, for both staff and the relatives of other patients, there is a psychological benefit in the stability of their presence.

However short their stay, staff become very attached to patients; and it is comforting for them too to be able to nurse someone who will be with them for longer. However, some question whether hospices are the right place for such patients themselves, as they must bear the added pain of regularly seeing people die to whom they have grown attached.

One exception to the hospice norm of caring mainly for cancer patients is St Joseph's Hospice in East London. The largest of all in-patient units, it has 125 beds. Fifty are for cancer patients. The remainder are for people who are chronically sick or physically handicapped.

~~

CHILDREN AS PATIENTS

Hospices do not, as a rule, take children as patients. As one medical director put it: "We don't think we know enough about caring for children and the paediatric dosage for drugs. We feel that the majority will be better at home or in a busy paediatric ward, rather than in a hospice with a large proportion of elderly patients." But the same doctor also admitted that occasionally, when it did seem appropriate, his hospice had indeed taken a family with a dying child, caring for him or her in a single ward.

Given a choice, most families would probably prefer to

care for their child at home, with the support of their own general practitioner. There is, however, one hospice called Helen House in Oxford which specialises in the care of dying children, and also children with long-term illnesses for which there is no cure. Its aim is to help to make it possible for families to care for their children themselves, at home, most of the time, in the knowledge that Helen House is there for occasional respite from the physical and emotional strain of coping, and for expert symptom control and family support. It is a bright and beautiful place, designed and furnished with children in mind, and has room for eight children plus parents to stay at any one time.

Not all those involved in the care of the dying feel that children should be segregated from general hospice care, however. There is now a movement based in the USA, called Children's Hospice International, which aims to support any hospice that adds a few beds for very young people. They believe that caring for young and old together can, in fact, bring rewards for both.

~

CATCHMENT AREAS

It has been estimated that to provide hospice-type care for all who may need it across the country, would require 45-50 in-patient beds per million of the population, and a minimum of four home care nurses per million. Very sadly, a great many regions fall far short of that, which inevitably means that people in some parts of the country will not have access to any hospice care. (The Hospice Information Service can provide details of hospice care available in all areas. The address appears on page 120.)

Hospices do, on the whole, take people only from within their own catchment area. This isn't just a bureaucratic ruling. Because family support is so vital a feature of

33

WHOM CAN HOSPICES HELP?

hospice caring, it doesn't make sense for a patient to be transported far away from home, to a place where friends and family cannot travel regularly and with ease. But no hospice would be so hardhearted as not to consider a justifiable exception. For instance, if a parent lived alone in Devon but children and grandchildren lived in London, it might be possible for care to be given in a hospice where it was easier for them to visit.

PAYING FOR HOSPICE CARE

Even though many hospices are independently funded, or only partly funded by the National Health Service, no one need ever worry that treatment and care in hospices must be paid for by the patient or family.

A very few hospices do have to ask for a contribution, and certainly all welcome donations to support their work, but money is not what decides admission. If a patient has private health insurance, however, the insurance will be claimed, so that the money can be used to contribute to general hospice running costs.

IN-PATIENT OR HOME CARE?

Finally, it is worth saying that no one form of care is invariably right for everyone. It is very often said that the best place to die is at home, and this is indeed the wish of a great many people who have loving relatives who are able to care for them there. It is, as mentioned above, towards more home care services that the hospice movement as a whole is directing its development; more

34

people can be helped, and in the setting that suits them best.

But there are others who, however caring and willing their relatives, cannot bear to be a burden, or who would prefer that their more intimate physical needs were carried out by nurses. Some families may just not have the facilities to cope, the adults may not be able to take leave from their jobs, or perhaps the dying person has no friends or family at all. For these, the in-patient units have much to offer.

And there are others again, particularly younger people, who may well prefer to remain in hospital having every possible treatment on offer, however remote the chance of success, rather than to spend their last days in a hospice where the emphasis is on comfort but not on cure.

Hospices do not set themselves up to be superior to everyone and everything else in matters of death and dying. But they are there, with their specialist skills and experience and almost awesome human compassion, for as many of those who want them as they can help.

3.

WHAT ARE HOSPICES LIKE?

Hospices share a common philosophy of caring, but they are each very individual places indeed.

It is probably true to say that no two are quite alike. Some have only eight or ten beds and so are extremely homely. Others, while doing their utmost to achieve as homelike an atmosphere as possible, are catering for 50 to 60 patients at a time. Some hospices are purpose-built, others have to make the best of whatever environment they have inherited. Some strike the visitor first as lively, laughing, active places, others exude an atmosphere of peace and ease.

Whatever the individual differences, some of which may reflect the personalities and approach of the particular people in charge, all strive to achieve one quality in common — a sense of safety, openness and freedom from tension, which arises from the nature of hospice-style care itself.

ATMOSPHERE AND AMENITIES

For those who have never been inside a hospice, I shall try to describe the kind of ambience they aim for, allowing, of course, for all possible individual variations.

Many hospices have been purpose-built. They are likely to be light and bright, with plenty of windows looking out over well cared-for and interestingly laid-out gardens. Whether purpose-built or not, there will probably be flowers and luscious-leaved green plants brightening the reception, the stairways, the sitting rooms and balconies as well as the wards. Walls are not institution green or cream, but are painted in the subtle shades that people choose for their own houses; and they are likely to be enlivened by paintings that hold the eye. Everywhere that can be will be comfortably carpeted.

What a hospice offers in terms of social amenities will obviously depend upon its size and its wealth. Some have several sitting rooms for patients and their relatives, with comfortable places to sit and relax, or to sit and write. Some may boast a bar and a library.

The larger hospice may have special areas set aside as out-patient clinics and as day centres. The large, bright, airy wards will probably be divided into separate bays of four beds to create a more intimate atmosphere.

There is no unpleasant, institutional smell, nor is the eye struck by the more usual accoutrements of hospital care — nurses busying about with thermometers or kits to test blood pressure, and doctors with stethoscopes slung around their necks. Dame Cicely Saunders always used to say that a pretty necklace was much better for a patient to look at than a stethoscope.

In a hospice, there is not the emphasis on the routine monitoring that goes on automatically in hospitals, but all the necessities for medical and nursing care are still there. This includes, when necessary, access to facilities for radiotherapy or surgery, when such intervention can ease unpleasant symptoms for a patient.

Many people, on seeing a hospice for the first time, are amazed by the relaxed and easy-going atmosphere that seems to permeate everywhere. Used, perhaps, to the hospital ward, where patients are neatly arranged in their beds and everything has to fit around a sacrosanct system, it is a surprise to see so many supposedly extremely seriously ill people walking and sitting around, fully dressed.

"We always encourage people to get up and dressed, if they can," said one hospice nurse, "because it is so good for morale, for the way they see themselves." When all someone has to do is to put on a coat, it no longer seems as if a superhuman effort has to be made just to go outside and enjoy the sun and flowers for a while.

~

SMOKING AND DRINKING

Habits, albeit bad ones, are not necessarily frowned on. People who smoke, for instance, can usually carry on smoking in the hospice; and no one is discouraged from having an alcoholic drink. On the contrary, in some hospices, a drink is routinely offered before dinner, as an aperitif helps to make mealtimes more of an occasion.

~

FOOD

Never, in hospices, should unappetising meals be served up in unappetising dollops plonked on a plate. The social and emotional significance of food is taken into account. Eating together can bring families closer, while a patient's loss of appetite can cause concern to the family, as well as the patient.

Sometimes relatives feel guilt and a sense of shame if a patient, who refused to eat at home, suddenly starts tucking into hospice meals with relish. But it should be remembered that pain and other symptoms of physical discomfort all affect appetite; once these symptoms are expertly controlled by the hospice doctor, appetite may spontaneously surge back.

The hospice menu does not offer up invalid food. The prevailing philosophy is that a little of what people fancy does them good, and quite often that is fish and chips! There is usually as wide a choice as possible, and special tastes or special requirements (e.g. vegetarian, or choices based on religious or cultural grounds) are catered for.

Portions are always attractively served, and are likely to be small — it can be dispiriting for patients to see so much food left over on their plate, even after they have eaten what they feel is a lot. Meal times are not rushed, and those who are embarrassed to need help to feed themselves, or who need to be fed, can be sure that they will be offered all due privacy.

Meal times are not rigid either. Those still asleep when breakfast is served are likely to be offered the chance to have it later. In other words, everything is as natural and homelike as possible.

ACTIVITIES

Always, the accent is on *living*, and different hospices offer what they can, in their different ways and in accordance with their own individual ideas. One hospice may arrange occasional candle-lit suppers or teas out on the lawn. Another may organise coach outings, for those who are well enough, to places of interest or the surrounding countryside.

At one hospice, once a week, children of the staff come in and sing, or someone sits at the piano and leads staff and patients in good old rousing sing-songs. I myself have been a member of a storytelling troupe booked for an occasional evening's entertainment at another hospice. Relatives, staff and patients all came to hear, and the stories sparked off many long-forgotten and fondly recalled reminiscences.

In very many hospices, it is quite common for the men at least to enjoy going off to the pub — and if they need to be accompanied by a nurse, the nurse will never be in uniform. Whatever wish a person may have is honoured if practically possible. There is a moving story of a young woman patient at Countess Mountbatten House, a Macmillan continuing care unit in Southampton, who looked out at the snow from the window of the ward and wished she could feel the cold, clean air on her face just one more time. She was wrapped up very warmly and taken outside in her bed, for that last strong yearning to be fulfilled and, consequently, to be recalled with considerable pleasure up until the time, some while later, that she died.

Whatever the request, it is in the spirit of hospice care to try and meet it, because emotional and spiritual needs are seen to be just as important as physical ones. One hospice sister said: "If a patient keeps saying he misses the cat or he would love a pint at his local or he wants to see his roses in bloom, no matter how ill he is, we will make it possible for him to go, if he really wants to."

Sometimes, though, relatives' unfounded fears have first to be put at rest. The same sister said: "We had one elderly lady here who very quickly started to bloom once we had her symptoms under control. She started talking wistfully of visiting her home again (she had a husband but he was very deaf and couldn't care for her on his own). We felt she could go for a weekend, but it was her son who proceeded to protest. It was as if he had adjusted in his mind to the fact that she was dying and couldn't see that her need right now was to carry on living. He was frightened that, if she went home, she would lose the hospice bed. But that would never happen. We always keep the bed for a patient home on a visit."

—∾—

OTHER THERAPIES

Although hospices do not offer curative medical treatments, people do not have to know or accept that they are dying in order to enter one, nor do they have to have given up all hope of any miracle themselves.

It is human to hope, and no hopes are ever quashed, although neither are illusions fostered. "But if someone has a belief in the power of certain herbs or in some particular diet or therapy, we will do our best to respect that belief and make them available," said a nurse. For there is no one set of beliefs so entrenched in the philosophy of hospice care that it cannot take on board a patient's own, whatever they may be.

4.

THE HOSPICE TEAM

The hospice's most important resource is, of course, the people who work there. Because of the demanding and intimate nature of the work, and the small size of hospices compared with hospitals, they operate very much as a team.

Again, depending upon the size of the unit, some or all of the following people will have a place on the caring team: doctors, nurses, social workers, physiotherapists, occupational therapists, chaplain and volunteers. Also very vital in the role they perform are the clerical, catering and cleaning staff who have contact with the patients.

CHOOSING STAFF

Staff who are going to work with dying patients are very
carefully chosen indeed. Not only must they be skilled in
their own particular profession, but their motivation for
wanting to work in a hospice has to be carefully examined.
Someone who has himself or herself lost someone close
within the previous two years may well not be strong
enough yet to offer others the necessary support in grief.
Because the emotional demands in a hospice are high, it is
also essential for staff to have supportive family or friends,
outside of their work and colleagues.

Compassion and caring are, of course, vital, but
individuals who are drawn towards working with the dying
because of the strength and zealousness of their own
religious convictions are not necessarily the most suitable
candidates; they may find it hard or upsetting to deal with
patients who have no religious beliefs of their own.

Conversely, someone who believes that there is no real
meaning to life, and that death is the end of everything,
may find it hard not to succumb to the stress that dying
and bereavement bring. As one fulfilled hospice nurse
said: "There is less stress for us here than you might
expect because we work and support each other as a team
and none of us believes that death in itself is a
catastrophe."

SHARING TASKS

As a team, there are not the strict demarcation lines
between duties which might more usually be found
elsewhere. Everyone is willing to do bits of each other's
job, as and when appropriate. And it is always the
patient's own choice whom he or she wishes to talk to

most intimately. It may be one doctor, but not the other who also does rounds on that ward; it may be the sister in charge, or the auxiliary nurse who helps the patient in the bath.

~

DOCTORS

The doctor's particular and most important role is that of diagnosis, eliciting the cause of distressing symptoms, prescribing drugs or whatever is appropriate to remedy them, and monitoring their use. This is a very specialised area indeed (symptom control will be dealt with fully in the next chapter).

The hospice doctor, however, will always have time to talk, and is not in the least remote in the way that, so often, hospital consultants are perceived to be. They are ready to offer comfort, to dispel worries with accurate information when requested, or just to listen to whatever a patient or a relative wants to say.

Doctors are seen on the wards almost as often as the nurses; they are on hand as needed 24 hours a day, and muck in with everyone else as required. They do not see themselves as more important than other members of the team, but purely as having their own special expertise in a particular area, just as their colleagues do.

~

NURSES

Nurses very often choose to work in hospices because they want to have the time to get to know dying patients and their needs, and offer them every comfort of nursing care.

This is something that is almost an unknown luxury in busy overstretched National Health Service hospitals. In hospices, nurses are in a very high ratio to patients, so they can willingly and gladly pay attention to all the little details that add up to making people feel comfortable, cossetted and cared for, as well as all the more obvious aspects of care.

For instance, however much easier and quicker it might be for nurses to wash a patient in bed, that is never the rationale for doing so. Because taking a bath or a shower is a pleasure, even if help is required for it, this will be encouraged for as long as is possible, and the pleasure may be enhanced with bubble bath or bath oil.

The nurse will know to pay attention to details such as making sure a bedridden patient is turned every couple of hours to prevent bedsores, and is prepared to spend an age bolstering up pillows until they are just right to provide adequate support. As patients who can sit in chairs are still at risk of pressure sores, they too will be remembered and be encouraged to shift position or take a walk at frequent intervals.

Mouth care is seen as routinely important, as thrush is very common in the seriously ill and causes additional distress. Also, if someone's mouth feels dry or not fresh, that can significantly affect their appetite. Mouth care is never neglected, however near a person is to death. If toothpaste or toothbrushing are not practical, there are always alternatives such as mouthwashes, or even flavoured ice cubes.

Nothing that a patient needs or might benefit from, for comfort, is ever seen as too much trouble for hospice nurses, and they will always do their imaginative and thoughtful best.

AUXILIARIES

Most hospices will have on their staff not only trained nurses but a number of untrained nurses called auxiliaries to help with basic nursing care. Although they are untrained, they often have a great deal of personal experience, because they are likely to work in a hospice for a number of years and become the mainstays of a ward.

Auxiliaries are taught not only basic nursing skills but how to behave in their personal dealings with patients. It may well be to an auxiliary, for instance, during bath time, that patients hint for the first time of their fears or worries about whether they are dying. They may, indeed, be asking the auxiliary rather than the doctor or sister in charge because they are not yet ready to hear the whole truth. Auxiliaries, along with everyone else, will be taught never to lie or offer false hope, but always to stay with patients at their own pace, and not give too much information too soon or, conversely, too little.

It might be felt that the auxiliaries and nurses, who are with their patients all day and all night, have to become immured to grief and detach themselves emotionally in order to carry on. Nothing could be further from the truth. All hospice staff become involved with their patients as people because otherwise they couldn't relate to them with real understanding. As one nurse said: "We aren't hardened. We do each get attached to certain patients. Perhaps we may break down and cry when reading a prayer by the bed of a patient who has just died. It is good for that chink in our armour to be seen, by relatives and other patients. We are only humans, after all."

SOCIAL WORKERS

Not all hospices have a full-time social worker on their staff, but there is usually someone who comes in at least part-time to help to sort out a whole host of problems that may face patients or their relatives. (They often play even more of a role in the home care team, which will be described in a later chapter.)

Firstly, the social worker is usually the person who tries to deal with any practical problems, such as financial difficulties or unfinished business that is worrying a patient, or the acquiring of grants to meet the patient's and relatives' needs when a patient goes home. Such things might include arranging a night sitter, arranging for a telephone to be installed in a patient's home, acquiring a grant to cover a family member's travelling expenses to visit, in a case of dire need, or getting something done about a faulty heating system.

Secondly, there may be many concerns of an emotional nature troubling a patient which a social worker can help to resolve. Often, for instance, when patients learn they are very ill and faced with the loss of their independence and, eventually, the loss of their life, many painful previous losses may come back to flood their consciousness as well: a divorce, perhaps, or a miscarriage years ago not fully grieved over at the time. These kinds of sorrows can be skilfully coaxed out into the open by the social worker, and the pain of their experience worked through.

Sometimes patients may suffer secret fears about what will happen to the look of their body, or how their loved ones will feel seeing them deteriorate, or how their loved ones will cope if they themselves become increasingly irritable and demanding. These kinds of fears might perhaps be mentioned in passing to a nurse, and the nurse may feel that the patient could benefit from the social worker's understanding, reassurance and support.

Often, too, terrific tension may be experienced within

families faced by something so seemingly catastrophic as a dear one's death. Old grievances and ensuing guilt, or misplaced over-zealousness to protect the dying person from any ordinary day-to-day family problems (thus unintentionally making them feel useless or worthless) may create a barrier between family members at a time when they most want and need to be close. The social worker will be alerted to these kinds of problems and, if it is helpful arrange a family meeting to try to deal with them.

PHYSIOTHERAPISTS

People are often surprised to learn that physiotherapists have a role in hospices at all. They associate them with rehabilitation, and what, after all, is the point of that if a person is dying? There is much point, and those hospices which do have the services, full-time or part-time, of a physiotherapist consider themselves fortunate.

The aim of physiotherapy is not to put patients through a set routine of uncomfortable gymnastics designed to be "good" for them, but to adapt what physiotherapy has to offer in order to encourage the patients' own independence for as long as this is possible. It may be the physiotherapist who suggests that someone shaky on their feet after a long period in bed tries to walk again, and who stands by to offer encouragement and help, generating confidence that walking will indeed be possible again.

It may be the physiotherapist who assesses the strength in an arm or a hand and recommends the use of particular gadgets, such as a special fork with the cutting edge of a knife, so that patients are still able to feed themselves.

Learning simple breathing exercises, to prevent infections developing in the lungs, and other types of exercises designed to increase mobility in a joint, can help

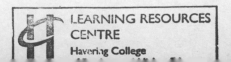

to create both a sense of achievement and, with the experience of improvement itself, purpose and great determination.

Simple massage may do much to relieve discomfort and pain, not only because it stimulates the circulation but also because the touch of loving, caring hands is a tonic in itself.

Physiotherapy in a hospice is essentially about relieving discomfort and, by removing some physical limitations, also removing the mental limitations patients may impose on themselves. It is easy to start thinking, "I'm no good for anything any more", when it is becoming harder and harder to manage things for ourselves. Conversely, it is easier to recover a belief in our abilities and personal value when we can see physical signs of achievement.

There is not likely to be anything hale and hearty about the therapist's approach, but a simple sensitivity to each and every patient's own needs.

OCCUPATIONAL THERAPISTS

In a hospice there may well be some overlap between an occupational therapist's role and that of a physiotherapist. Both are concerned with helping a person make the most of *now*, rather than working towards a return to a previous lifestyle.

The occupational therapist may try to help patients recover or adapt some basic skills, such as shaving themselves or making a cup of coffee, so that they can feel confident about coping again at home. Another important task is to help stretch patients' sense of their own achievement, encouraging them perhaps to paint, or to make small handicrafts as gifts, the giving of which may bring much pleasure.

But great care is taken to gear any such work or leisure activities to the needs of the individuals themselves, their interests and their sense of themselves as people. Whatever patients do embark on doing must give *them* satisfaction, rather than the staff! Occupational therapists often play their most important role in the running of the day unit, if the hospice has one, more of which will be said in Chapter 10.

~

CHAPLAINS

Some hospices may have a full-time chaplain, who can also call on the help of, say, a Catholic priest or a rabbi. Others may rely entirely upon volunteered services. The chaplain is there for those who need him. He does not force his attention upon those who don't. But it is often the case that, when people near death, they do turn back — or turn for the first time — to religion. The chaplain is then there, on call, to listen and to offer spiritual support of whatever kind is needed.

The chapel is an important place in a hospice, where staff and those patients who are able may go for prayers. If requested, the chaplain will say prayers for a family, or lead a funeral service. His is a very important role. Not only can he offer solid support to patients and relatives but also to the staff, whose spiritual needs, as human beings working with dying people, are just as great. He will not decide the terms on which people approach him, nor demand from them belief as he knows it, but will meet them and help them in whatever place they happen to be.

VOLUNTEERS

Volunteers in hospices are also very special people. Just as staff have to be chosen carefully, so do those who give their time free, for they too are an integral part of the hospice team. They need to have a joy in living, rather than a preoccupation with death. (Someone who has recently lost a loved one of their own is probably not ready to cope with the strong emotions of others.)

The volunteer must be able to talk and to listen, to support, to cope with the expression of strong and painful emotions, and not to judge others' lifestyles or beliefs. It is often, after all, to a volunteer who has come to be seen as a trusted friend, that a dying person chooses to reveal innermost feelings.

Volunteers' contribution to hospice care is wide-ranging. Some may take patients out for a ride in their cars, to the park or to visit a member of the family. They might take a patient to the opera or the theatre or, conversely, just sit by the bed of patients who have no visitors and hold their hand.

They may help with meals, make beds, and, for patients who have returned to be cared for at home, undertake night-sitting or do the daily shopping. Many become very skilled at supporting families in bereavement. A number of people who become volunteers are former nurses or other health professionals, but by no means all are.

It is perhaps important here to stress again that, while all care-giving groups in hospices have their own particular skills to offer, they are first and foremost part of a team in which those skills are shared. It may be that patients first choose to talk of their fears or anger not to the social worker, but to the physiotherapist who is massaging their back or the volunteer who is arranging their flowers. Or it may be to the occupational therapist who stops to bring them a glass of water or turns them to a more comfortable position.

There are no strict demarcation lines between what one professional considers it their "job" to perform and what another insists is theirs. All are offering whole care to a patient, as and how required, and relating to him or her as a human being.

5.

THE ROLE OF RELATIVES

INCLUDING THE FAMILY

A friend of mine was very wary, a year ago, when she was advised to let her mother go into a hospice. She had wanted to care for her at home but her mother was in some pain, and the strain and anxiety had become, at least for a while, too much.

Still, my friend felt that, by bringing her mother to the hospice, she would be seen as giving up on her, and would also cease to be able to play much personal part in her care. "The professionals are going to take over," she commented, somewhat bitterly, before admission.

The day after, she was a different person. "I can't believe what a wonderful place it is," she said. "It is so unlike anything I expected. I don't feel in the least bit shut out at all."

ON ARRIVAL

The personal and individualised quality of hospice care is noticeable instantly on arrival. At St Christopher's, for instance, to mention just one hospice, it is policy for a bed to be brought down and waiting in reception, with a hot water bottle already in it, ready for the new patient the moment they arrive. Matron will be standing alongside to greet both patient and relatives, and a nurse will be standing at the ward door specially, to say hullo as soon as they arrive upstairs.

Relatives are not made to feel, as soon as they reach the ward, that their presence is now redundant and even a nuisance. While the patient is settled in and made comfortable, they will be offered a cup of coffee, and given a chance to ask questions or voice any of their own anxieties.

Staff usually make a point of asking about any special likes and dislikes of a new patient. These will be noted down, so that Mrs Smith will continue to get the cup of tea and a biscuit she has always enjoyed before going to sleep, and Mr Jones will still have his watch wound for him and left where he can reach out to pick it up during the night.

There aren't usually any regimented rules about when a new patient must arrive. Arrivals are timed to suit families rather than staff. One man whose wife was scheduled to come into a hospice on a particular day mentioned regretfully that a family celebration had been planned for that night, and that his wife would dearly have liked to go. "Go by all means," said the hospice staff, "and just come along with her after." It didn't matter that, in the event, their actual arrival was delayed until about 1.30 in the morning.

Perhaps, for another family, it is important that the children can come along when grandma goes in, and so admission will be arranged for after school hours.

VISITING

All family members, including young children and family pets, are made welcome in a hospice. Relatives are positively encouraged not only to come but to help with the patient's care. As one hospice sister said: "Often relatives feel guilty if they can't do anything to help. They want to carry on participating in meeting the patient's needs. They don't want to feel useless, overtaken."

So it may be a husband or wife, or a daughter or nephew who helps their relative with their meals, with washing, with shaving, or who arranges the flowers. They may suggest sitting out in the gardens or going for a drive.

They are encouraged to contribute in any way they want to. If someone wants to bring in a special food that the patient loves, that is never seen as a slur on the skills of the kitchen staff.

YOUNG VISITORS

The presence of children, however young, is considered highly positive, but sometimes it is the hospice staff who have to persuade visiting relatives, and patients, to allow it. "Children really do cheer people up and, literally, bring them back from the grave," said a hospice nurse.

Sometimes, however, there are emotional barriers to be broken down first. A mother may think it will upset her young son to see grandad looking so frail and ill, or grandad himself may be reluctant for a treasured grandson to see him looking and behaving so differently from before.

It may take careful coaxing by the hospice staff to get the mother or grandfather to see that the child, if not allowed to visit, may imagine himself to be rejected; that

57

this story of grandad being too ill may be seen by him as
just a blind for the awful truth that really he isn't loved
any more — perhaps because of some minor
misdemeanour long forgotten by the adults involved, but
horribly alive in the child's mind.

~~

HOW MANY VISITORS?

In hospices there are no rules about how many people can
visit at one time, although common sense should obviously
prevail; too much stimulation may be very exhausting for
the patient. Relatives sometimes need to "learn" how to
visit, to realise that just sitting quietly by the bed, even if
nothing is said, is comforting to the patient, and certainly
more relaxing than a constant artificial attempt to keep
conversation going, or an insistence on well-meant,
distracting activities, such as playing cards.

Relatives can stay in the hospice for as long and as
often as they like, and usually there is some provision for
staying overnight whenever necessary.

~~

THE 'REST' DAY

There is, however, one day in the week — usually Monday
— when visiting is not allowed (unless, of course, a patient
is very close to death). Hospices generally have adopted
this rule for three important reasons.

Firstly, it is therapeutic for relatives to get used to how
it feels not being constantly in the dying person's
presence. Although their lives may be revolving entirely

around their loved one for the time being, they are going to have to pick up the threads of their own lives afterwards.

Having a day when visiting is not allowed also takes away any guilt a relative may feel about having a rest-day. Constant caring is too emotionally demanding and draining, and people need a break.

Thirdly, staff also want and need time to get to know their patients, and to offer them private time and a listening ear; it may be difficult for some patients to broach worries that are on their mind if their spouse is always by their side. Often it is hard to talk for the first time of sad or frightening things to someone that we love dearly, and it may take the intervention of an impartial but sympathetic third party to help us clear the way.

So the Monday no-visiting rule is not a meaningless convention, but a day's grace — designed, as with all things in hospices, to benefit both relatives and patients.

~~

RELATIVES AS PART OF THE CARE TEAM

In hospices, there is never a sense that relatives are a nuisance, and that everything could be much more cleanly and efficiently handled if they weren't around. Quite the contrary, as hospice consultant, psychiatrist Dr Murray Parkes, explained in an article in *The Management of Terminal Disease* (edited by Dr Cicely Saunders and published by Edward Arnold):

"In a terminal care ward, the patient's family are not intruders, nor are they honoured guests; they are an intimate part of the network of care. They are both care-givers and cared-for ... The patient's troubles are likely soon to be over, but the family's may be just beginning."

Much more will be said about the emotional needs of both patients and relatives in Chapter 7, so suffice it to say here that there is always some member of staff ready and willing to talk to relatives, at whatever time of day, about whatever concerns they may be feeling. Hospice care is quite firmly family-oriented.

6.

CONTROLLING SYMPTOMS

One of the greatest fears most of us probably still have about cancer is that someone who has it is going to die in terrible pain. In fact, according to statistics, to die of cancer is not necessarily a painful death — 40 per cent of people with very advanced cancer do not experience pain.

THE RELIEF OF PAIN

It is, however, very unfortunately true that a great many people with cancer suffer severe pain which *could* have been relieved, had someone only realised the need or known how to do it. It has been estimated that a fifth of cancer patients who die in hospital, and nearly a third of those who die at home, die in severe pain which it was not necessary for them to suffer.

There are a number of reasons why this is so. Very many hospital doctors and general practitioners do not know how to give effective pain relief in terminal illness. They may fear that if they prescribe substantial doses of narcotics, such as morphine, the patient will become addicted or immune to the effects. They also may not realise that the pain suffered is not always caused by the cancer itself, but may result from other kinds of discomfort, including emotional problems.

They may end up prescribing drugs that are too weak to work effectively, while the patients say nothing, either because they believe that cancer pain cannot be relieved, or because they are trying to disguise their pain, from their family or from facing it fully themselves.

It is a terrible thing to see a loved one in continuous pain, and that memory is one of the deepest scars that bereaved relatives carry with them. Fortunately, as hospice principles of care for the terminally ill become more widespread (not only in hospice in-patient units themselves, but in hospitals, and in support services for relatives caring for patients at home), unnecessary unrelieved cancer pain should eventually become a thing of the past.

ERASING THE MEMORY OF PAIN

Hospices are rightly famous for their skill in symptom control of every kind. A large proportion of their patients, on admission, are suffering severe pain; and all, very shortly afterwards, experience considerable and usually totally relief.

Effective symptom control is seen as the first task of hospice-style care because pain, particularly of an intense intermittent or chronic kind, blots out everything else and becomes the entire focus of a person's world. When suffering such pain, it is impossible to feel interested in anything else. It drains all energy and denies any positive feeling.

The first principle of pain relief used in hospices was learned by Dame Cicely Saunders, long before she became a doctor, from the nuns at St Luke's; and that is, to erase the memory of pain. We are used in our society to taking painkillers "as required", i.e. when the pain becomes too intrusive to bear. Such a regime has no place in the treatment of terminal pain. Only if the pain can be *anticipated* — that is, relief given before it makes itself felt again — can not only the experience of pain but the fear of pain be eliminated.

Many of us who dislike going to the dentist know that the anticipation of pain is often worse than what we really experience when we get there. And yet, how incomparable is that with the very real, severe pain that can be experienced with cancer, and the knowledge that agony must be endured at least for some while before the next painkilling dose, given "as required", relieves or perhaps merely reduces it.

In hospices, analgesics are normally given every four hours, at whatever dosage is required to eliminate pain, and to have an effect which will not yet have worn off by the time the next dose is due. In that way, the patient soon ceases not only to experience pain but even to remember the experience of pain.

It may not be necessary for a patient to be given a narcotic as an analgesic. Simpler remedies, such as aspirin or paracetamol, are very often adequate to relieve mild or moderate pain. Drugs of a kind usually used to treat arthritis can be very effective in relieving bone pain. But, if these do not have any effect, no hospice doctor would be fearful of prescribing a narcotic.

MORPHINE

In hospice care, the narcotic of choice is usually morphine, and the dosage may vary according to individual need — from 5 mg four-hourly to 150 mg, although the higher dosages are very rarely needed. One ill-founded belief which prevents many patients treated elsewhere from receiving adequate pain relief is that treatment with morphine will mean addiction. It is feared that the dosage will continually have to be increased to keep up. Eventually it will reach a ceiling where it has no pain-relieving effect at all, at a time, near the end, when the pain experienced may be the worst.

Long hospice experience has shown quite clearly that when morphine is taken by an ill person suffering severe pain, rather than by a healthy person seeking a high (heroin is diamorphine, morphine's equivalent), there are no addictive effects and the patient rarely develops tolerance to the dose. Only if *pain* increases will the dosage need to go up.

In fact, it is hospice experience that, as pain and the memory of pain fade, the dosage of morphine is more usually *lowered* than raised. Use of narcotics has been refined over the years in hospice care to achieve the simplest and most effective form of pain relief. For instance, they do not recommend the use of a once popular "cocktail" of drugs (still often used elsewhere) which includes alcohol and cocaine as well as morphine or heroin.

It is now felt that heroin offers no advantage over morphine, and that cocaine has no place because it can cause hallucinations and restlessness. The alcohol in the "cocktail" had such minimal effect that it is thought preferable, if patients want alcohol, for them to take it neat so that they can at least enjoy it!

It is also not considered good hospice practice routinely to combine morphine in a ready-made mixture with a drug that prevents nausea (often induced by narcotics), or a drug to act as a tranquilliser. Although both these additions may be necessary, if they are part of a ready-made mixture the proportion used necessarily increases along with the required proportion of morphine. Thus many patients may become over-sedated, and their mental faculties unnecessarily impaired, which is very distressing for themselves and for their relatives. The preferred practice is to give morphine diluted in chloroform water, which takes away the bitter taste, and to add anything else only as required.

Another benefit of giving morphine in solution is that the amount to be swallowed always remains the same, even if the proportion of morphine in it needs to be increased. Patients are therefore not forced to be aware each time medication is due that they are needing more pain relief than they did before.

Morphine injections are very rarely necessary, and are usually given only if a person cannot swallow or is semi-conscious.

~

CONTROLLING PHYSICAL DISCOMFORTS

Morphine is, however, only one member of the symptom control arsenal available for judicious use in hospices. Other kinds of discomfort may need completely different kinds of treatment. A whole range of drugs is available, to control nausea, vomiting, constipation, diarrhoea, loss of appetite, coughs, difficulty in breathing, insomnia etc.

Often relatives are frightened that the patient will suddenly haemorrhage, or choke, or have a fit. These kinds of emergencies are in fact rare when symptom control has been appropriate but, should they occur, there are still remedies available that can bring relief.

As a hospice doctor said: "No one is ever left feeling uncomfortable or in fear of what may happen." In fact, a feeling of safety is how so many patients — and their relatives — describe their own experience of hospice-style care.

~~

NON-PHYSICAL PAIN

But cancer pain is often far from entirely caused by physical symptoms. There may be a large psychological component as well which, if ignored, may well render fruitless all physical efforts to eliminate the pain.

Those who know they have a cancer that cannot be cured by medical means are only too likely to be anxious and fearful. They may feel a terrible rage and anger that this has happened to them. Unable to communicate their feelings to those closest to them, through fear of distressing them, or perhaps because of their relatives' own fear of causing distress, they can become increasingly isolated. In their mind they may go over their life and be filled with regrets for what was or was not; the anxiety may worsen the pain and, in its turn, bring on depression which exacerbates both.

Dame Cicely Saunders has defined four kinds of pain which may be experienced: physical pain; emotional pain (feeling helpless, isolated, angry etc.); social pain (worrying about how the family will react and cope afterwards); and spiritual pain (a longing to feel some purpose or meaning to life). In hospice care, attention is paid to all forms of pain. However, it is only after physical symptoms have been treated that a person may have the energy and space to get in touch with and tackle other equally crushing but less tangible promoters of pain. The total relief then experienced can be enormous.

Much more will be said about hospice-style handling of emotional pain in Chapter 7, but it should now be easier to understand why patients on morphine so often need less rather than more as time goes on. As fear and anxiety and all other kinds of emotional pain are brought out into the open and resolved, the need for physical forms of pain relief are lessened. And it is only in whole-person care, rather than symptom-oriented care, that opportunity for such significant relief is possible.

7.

EMOTIONAL NEEDS

When my mother, who had been a widow for many years, was diagnosed as having untreatable cancer of the oesophagus, my sister and I chose to care for her at home.

We were desperately upset, but we did feel confident about controlling the pain, and we expected to be able to talk honestly all together about what was happening, however much sadness it caused. The hospital doctor had been very sympathetic. When we asked if he had told our mother the truth, he said that he was always honest if he was asked by the patient, but that our mother hadn't asked.

She didn't ask us either. She didn't indicate that she knew she had cancer and talked of when she got better — although before she had gone into hospital, we knew that cancer had been the fear on her mind. We felt we couldn't deny her hopes or her will to fight, and so we involuntarily became caught up in the collusion of her recovery.

Emotionally, for us, it was an agonising time. Although we never ourselves encouraged her to think she was getting better, we felt, as time went on, that we let opportunities slip, when she might have been hinting for the truth, because of our own fear now, once having colluded, of not knowing how to act for the best.

Four years later, both my sister and I have very painful memories of the fact that, in the end, although we were both there, our mother may have been left alone with unvoiced fears, or with feelings she wanted to share with us. We still wish we had had access to the kind of emotional help that hospice staff so expertly offer.

Many of us have, no doubt, sometimes tried to imagine how we would react if we learned that we or someone whom we loved had terminal cancer. The reality may be very different indeed. As my sister and I discovered, it can sometimes be very hard to break through the unanticipated barriers of fear, for all sorts of reasons. A last chance to be really close may then be lost.

But, equally important, how one chooses to die is the privilege of each individual, whether or not that fits the image the relatives would like. It is here that hospice staff are so very skilled in easing the way towards communication at the patient's own pace. No knowledge that the patients don't want is ever forced upon them, but neither are they ever deprived of honesty when it is asked for.

As matters of the emotions are rarely that black or white, of course, it may take considerable professional skill and understanding to identify and deal with the innumerable intervening shades of grey.

AVOIDING THE TRUTH

Both patients and relatives may have their own ways of

and reasons for avoiding open acceptance of the unlikelihood of cure. When patients first realise that they are likely to die, their reaction is very often one of complete shock and numbness, an inability to absorb such an overwhelming discovery and, therefore, a denial that it has happened. The denial may in part be a way to block out having to face frightening thoughts about what the immediate future may hold — loss of independence, increasing feelings of debility, fear for the family's future without them, and so on.

Denial can take various forms. Patients may refuse to talk about anything which might lead on to uncomfortable thoughts or discussions about illness or death. They may, however, start to feel increasingly anxious, but claim that they have no idea at all what they have to feel so anxious about. Alternatively, they may seemingly accept the truth, but at a much deeper level feel totally unable to allow it to sink in.

Sometimes, for instance, patients may ask about and be told the truth about their condition, and then apparently instantly forget what they have heard. They may ask again the next day, and the next, and each time react as if they were hearing it for the first time. Unconsciously they may feel that they *should* be strong enough to cope with the truth, but in fact, emotionally, they aren't yet ready for it. Behaving as we think we ought or as we think befits our sense of dignity or status is often counter-productive because it conflicts with basic, universal emotions such as fear.

Dr Murray Parkes has written of a middle-aged woman who came into St Christopher's Hospice for symptom control. She had insisted that her doctor tell her the truth and also insisted that she had no fear of dying. But she was upset to see when she looked in the mirror that her face had a permanent look of terror, with her eyelids retracted in fear. This did not square with her intellectually chosen stance of having no fear of death. Only when she could allow herself to accept help did the fear diminish and her face relax.

Sometimes people who persist in denying the seriousness of their illness or their concern about it do so because in the past they have been deeply affected by the death of someone close to them, and did not fully express their sadness or fear at the time.

Another quite common form of denial is to experience fear or concern, but not on one's own behalf. A man may say that he has adjusted to the idea that he is dying and that all his concern is for what will happen to his wife. He may make her extremely anxious and confused by the overly strong concern he expresses on her behalf and, unintentionally, both become distanced from each other.

A state of numbness may at some point give way to a state of anxiety, or bitterness and anger at the unfairness and unreasonableness of it all. The anger has to be expressed somehow. However, instead of being acknowledged for what it is, it very often gets vented on hospital staff or relatives. This can be particularly painful for relatives, of course, if the reasons are not understood.

THE FEARS OF RELATIVES

It may be difficult for relatives to know how to react to these sorts of responses, especially if they are struggling alone, without the benefit of help from professionals who themselves are comfortable in dealing with the emotional needs of dying patients. But there is often the added difficulty that relatives, too, may unconsciously deny their own fears about death and the loss of a loved one.

There is just as likely to be unfaced fear, for instance, when it is the relative who insists that he or she is all right, and that the only person they should be concerned about is the patient. Or when a husband or wife says that there is surely no point in discussing the true diagnosis with the patient, as it will only increase distress.

It is natural to be fearful about what will happen to a loved one, what pain or discomfort they might have to experience, what physical changes they may go through, such as loss of weight and energy and mental alertness. Such fears are likely to be even stronger if someone else in the past was seen to die painfully from cancer, because they may believe then that all such deaths are the same. These fears may well, in fact, be unnecessary, but they cannot be assuaged if they are not acknowledged.

It is also natural, even if the thought is pushed away as too frightening or too horribly selfish, to worry about what is going to happen to oneself, left alone and empty after a partner or a beloved parent or only child has died.

Relatives very often fear that the loved one who is dying won't be able to cope with the enormity of knowing the truth. They may be frightened of causing a sadness so engulfing, both in themselves and in the dying person, that they will not be able to offer sufficient comfort.

Some may fear that the truth will hasten death in a loved one because they will lose all will to carry on living. It is also true that people who learn they have incurable cancer do sometimes have fleeting or not so fleeting thoughts of suicide, and telling the truth is sometimes avoided for fear that this will be the result.

All of these kinds of fears, if they are suppressed, may cause more pain to all concerned than the pain of sharing. But it demands great courage to take what seems an enormous risk and share these fears. That is where it may help so much to have the skilled and sympathetic assistance of impartial but caring third parties.

COMMON ANXIETIES

Much has been written by professionals and researchers in hospice care, here and abroad, about the emotional aspects of death for both patients and relatives.

Psychiatrist Dr Colin Murray Parkes, who has been published most extensively on the subject, found, in his researches, that the most common fears expressed by patients with terminal cancer are those of being separated from the people they love, the home they know and the jobs they may have done for years. They fear, in other words, abandonment and loss of identity.

Also common are anxieties about loss of physical and mental control, and becoming a burden to others. Some fear that they will not be able to achieve a particular goal they had set their hearts on, or that an obligation which hangs over them will remain unfulfilled.

The prospect of death in the not too distant future is perhaps particularly difficult to accept when a person has remained in an unsatisfactory relationship, with both partners clinging to the hope that things will improve when the awaited job comes through, or they can move to the country, or the children are off their hands, or whatever. Suddenly, what has gone before seems like so much time lost; it appears that there will be no future now to make the sacrifices worthwhile.

~

THE BENEFITS OF BEING OPEN

These kinds of fears are likely to be felt in some form, even if patients have not consciously acknowledged their physical condition, or if their relatives refuse openly to do so. If it is the relatives who, in their fear of inducing insufferable mental pain, avoid honest communication with the patient, the patient may be denied many opportunities to keep a degree of control over their own life and involvement in that of their family. Thus, indeed, the common fear of patients that they will be abandoned and lose their sense of identity may unintentionally be realised, because of a lack of openness.

Patients may want to use what time they have left to make provisions for their family. They may want to make or change a will, or to give certain gifts during their lifetime. They may want to plan ahead for the education of their children, or tie up business affairs, or complete some important or cherished project, or repair an old rift with a brother unseen for years.

Families may think they are being kindest by keeping patients in the dark and sparing them any additional burdens, such as knowledge of mounting bills, or some problem with a wayward adolescent at school. In fact, however, they may be leaving the patients in a state of unconfirmed suspicion, and depriving them of feeling a sense of mastery over aspects of their life, such as participating in or making family decisions.

For such reasons, among others, Swiss-born Dr Elisabeth Kubler Ross, one of the pioneers of caring work with the dying in the United States, believes that knowing the truth about his or her condition should be the patient's choice, and the patient's alone.

~

COMING TO TERMS WITH DEATH

For those who would choose to know, knowing also has other advantages. Patients have the chance to come to terms with their own death and what it means to them, emotionally and spiritually. And, in the honest sharing of the truth with loved ones, there is the chance for free and open communication between them, a chance to express their true feelings, to right old nagging wrongs and to face each new development with shared concern — instead of being separated by divisive secrecy, false cheerfulness and fear.

Researchers have found that patients with untreatable

cancer who are aware of and can accept their condition, and who have close support from people they love, tend to live for longer than might otherwise have been expected.

Dame Cicely Saunders has written of a patient who asked her to tell him the truth and, when she did, said: "Thank you. It is hard to be told but it is hard to tell too. Thank you." It is very, very hard for a relative to have to be the one to tell (and the relative may not be the best person to do so); but hiding the truth may bring health risks of its own for the relatives. For instance, the horror of knowing something so momentous yet keeping it hidden from his loved one, or the fear of facing life without her, may mean a husband stops himself from taking in what the doctors tell him. He may then be unprepared for his wife's death when it does happen, and the shock, coupled with repressed anxiety and tension, can precipitate a breakdown.

It is with all these kinds of conflicting emotional needs and fears that hospice professionals know how to help.

8.

TALKING ABOUT DYING

"We do not stand over people and say, 'You *do* realise you are dying, don't you?' We let people unfold and we move at their pace," said a hospice sister.

Hospices aim for an atmosphere of security, openness and trust. Patients are made to feel welcomed and wanted. Once symptoms, which may have been crippling or frightening them for weeks, have been controlled, they can start to feel safe and relaxed. There is no secretive whispering of staff at the end of the bed, nor is there a whirlwind of thermometer shaking and blood pressure testing that makes people feel the staff must be far too busy to have any time to talk.

On the contrary, all staff make time to talk, sitting informally on the patients' beds if they aren't able to be up and about, or chatting side by side in chairs. The atmosphere itself is often enough to encourage people for the first time to broach concerns they have been keeping to themselves.

~~

CHOOSING WHOM TO TALK TO

It is up to patients to choose whom they want to talk to about anything. Just as anywhere else in life, we feel particularly drawn to or safe with one person rather than another. Some may choose to express their worries to the doctor, others may suddenly ask something of the nurse who is helping with their bath. Some patients may only ever talk openly to the volunteers who take them out for a drive, because they see them as just "ordinary" people like themselves.

People who work in hospices are individuals who have their own ways of encouraging a patient to discuss any fears, or reacting to direct questions. There is no mystique about it. Their skill comes from experience, from empathy, from being able to trust their own judgments and, very importantly, from a basic respect for another human being's needs and rights.

Honesty is the key, but so is the principle of giving neither more nor less information than a person wants to know. A doctor may talk to patients about their physical condition, and wait and see whether the patients themselves take the conversation on to ask about their future. The doctor may well ask "Do *you* have anything you would like to talk about with me?", so that patients know that the time and the concern are available if they want to talk.

Even if a hospice has been told by a patient's hospital doctor or general practitioner that the patient "knows", staff will not presume that they can instantly be open. The patient may indeed have been told, but has also "forgotten" — being not yet ready to cope. Questions that seem to demand a direct answer, such as "I'm not going to get better, am I?" may be answered first with another question (e.g. "What makes you think that?"), so that it is possible to gauge from what is then said how much a person really wants to know.

～

GRADUAL ACCEPTANCE

There may be many stages of truth-telling. Some who come into a hospice for symptom control may be able to carry on living almost normally at home for a good while after, once distressing discomfort has been relieved. It may be appropriate for them to come to terms with their gradually changing condition little by little, accepting first the fact that they may be unable to carry on their job, later that they may not be able to move around very easily or that they won't have the energy for certain activities they used to enjoy. Much later may come the acceptance that the time left to them is limited.

According to hospice staff, very many people do not ask outright if they are dying, or directly express their own knowledge that they are. Some may ask instead if there will be any pain, or what will happen to a pet. How and what people ask dictate the nature of the answers.

Sometimes, patients who yesterday wanted reassurance that their death would be peaceful, or who were talking peaceably about feeling calm and ready to die, whenever it happened, are the following day discussing plans for next year, or even ten years' time. That may be upsetting or confusing to relatives, but it is not unfamiliar to hospice workers.

It can be quite a positive thing not to want to think all the time about death, but rather to acknowledge it and then push it out of the way, so as to carry on living the moment right now. It is quite common, in hospice experience, for people to be able to hold two conflicting ideas, that of awareness of likely imminent death, and that of having hopes or plans for the future and deriving enjoyment from them.

~~

A DIRECT ANSWER

Those who do seek a very direct answer are not denied one. For instance, patients may be thinking of buying a new house, or just about to embark on a new business venture, or have the desire to see a distant relative before they die. If they ask if it would be sensible to forget the house or the business venture, or if they should make plans to see the relative as soon as possible, they will be given an honest answer.

One question that is usually impossible to answer, however, is "How long have I got?" How long will depend on so many things, including how widespread the cancer is, what kinds of treatment have gone before, the age of the patient, the support given by family and friends, and the patient's own attitude towards life and death.

~~

REQUESTS NOT TO TELL

Very often, relatives beg hospice staff not to tell patients that they are dying. It is a request that is born of fear, for all the variety of aforementioned reasons, and cannot be granted. The hospice's duty is to tell a patient all that he or she expresses a wish to know, and to support them through it. But the relatives will be supported too, and helped to see that this way is for the best.

One woman who was suffering from breast cancer was brought into a hospice without having any idea of what was the matter with her. Her doctor had been evasive, and her relatives were frightened. They asked the sister in charge not to tell her the truth.

But, after a few days, the woman herself became aware that people around her seemed to be very ill. She said to a young nurse, whom she particularly liked, "These people look as if they have cancer. Do I have cancer?" She was in considerable distress, and put a lot of pressure on the young nurse. The sister advised the nurse to sit on the woman's bed and tell her the truth.

Afterwards the woman was very upset. She cried for a long time and became depressed. When her relatives came to visit her and found her this way, they too became very upset and also very angry.

"What they didn't understand then was that it is very therapeutic for people to feel sad and depressed when they learn that they are dying," said the hospice sister. "It is only normal to feel sad when we receive bad news. We always spend a lot of time with a patient when they have been told. We reassure them that they can be here as long as they like and talk to anyone they choose, the medical director, the social worker, whomever, at any time they like. They realise they will not be left alone and need keep no worries to themselves.

"The sadness lasts a few days and then they really swim up. It's amazing how the stress just suddenly falls off both the patient and the relatives afterwards."

The sadness is seen as something natural that needs to be experienced first, however distressing it may appear to others. For that reason, the prescription of anti-depressants in such circumstances is not encouraged.

HELP WITH TELLING THE TRUTH

Relatives are very often frightened of being asked themselves by their loved one if he or she is dying. Answering is an awesome responsibility, and the fear can helpfully be shared with the hospice doctor or matron, who will be able to offer expert advice, especially as they will themselves have a sense of what particular patients do and do not want to know. One hospice sister said: "We try to help relatives to relax, and tell them not to rehearse what they think they will say, if asked, but to try to be truthful if they can."

Very often, though, one of the benefits of hospice care is that the staff are there to ease the way for painful communication between patient and family. Just as often as a husband is fearful of being truthful to his wife about her condition, so is she fearful of letting him know what she already knows herself but fears he couldn't handle. It may well be the case that both people know and know each other knows, yet cannot bring themselves to voice that knowledge.

The social worker may be the one who can talk with patients about their feelings, and about whether they would like to communicate these to their spouse or children. If patients want to but cannot bring themselves to be the one to broach the subject, they may agree that the social worker should tell the family what has been said between them. They may even arrange a meeting at which the social worker is also present to help open the way to acknowledgment and sharing.

9.

SUPPORT FOR RELATIVES

For very many relatives of a patient in a hospice, it is their first experience of losing someone close. They may have numerous fears or beliefs which are in fact unfounded, but they will not be left to flounder with these alone. Just as hospice staff are skilled at helping patients feel comfortable and safe enough to talk, so are they skilled at understanding the needs of relatives. They will offer information, encourage discussion, and sense when their support is or is not appropriate.

Straightforward things, such as discussing with the nearest relatives every change in the patient's condition and what this is likely to mean now and in the near future, can help to put troubled minds at rest. Someone who has never seen anyone die before may fear that death will be painful, or not peaceful, or very sudden, none of which may be the case. Or they may need help to realise that the patient who seems to look so different from the robust or lively person they loved is still the same person underneath, and still has the same feelings and needs.

OFFERING INFORMATION

Many hospices make a point of offering information rather than waiting to be asked.

Often people have worries which they fear will be laughed at, or which they are too embarrassed to mention. Some partners, for instance, will find it difficult to ask whether, when a patient is coming home, it will be all right to continue their sex life. Or they may secretly wonder if cancer is catching. (It isn't.)

PATIENTS' EMOTIONAL NEEDS

Very many families welcome the support and understanding of staff in cases when the patient becomes angry towards them, or seemingly listless and uninterested in life. Certain patients have to go through these stages in their acceptance of death, but they can cause intense pain to the unprepared family.

Close family members may also have important information to *give* hospice staff which will help them in their care of a patient. If, for instance, someone remains very depressed for a long time after learning that they are dying, it may be because they have suffered from depression intermittently throughout their lives; as a result they may well benefit from an anti-depressant, since the sadness in such a case is unlikely to lift on its own.

When someone is dying, their needs and perceptions are ever-changing. To appreciate this, it may be helpful to have the assistance of people who are outside the family — especially as what a caring relative and what the patient perceives as a need may in fact differ. As already mentioned, relatives may consider it a sensible kindness to spare patients from involvement in the day-to-day ups and downs of family affairs, at a time when patients actually need to feel wanted and still worthwhile, and worthy of being listened to. There may come a stage, however, when their thoughts seem to revolve entirely around their condition and what is happening in their body, and relatives may feel hurt to find that they don't seem very interested in something they think is important.

~

A WORSENING CONDITION

Help may also be valuable in the transition between the time when patients are still relatively independent and deriving mental strength from their own physical achievement, and the time when they become reliant on others for their needs. They may dread losing control and becoming a burden; families may dread seeing them deteriorate, moving closer to death and thus, seemingly, further from them.

Yet, if these fears can be voiced and dispelled, the time of greatest need may turn out to be the most intimate time of all, both for the patients dying and for their loved ones. There is great intimacy indeed, in being allowed to give so much and allowing oneself to receive so much.

FAMILIES WITH CHILDREN

Much pain may be experienced on behalf of children, in the uncertainty of not knowing how to act for the best. It can help if the doctor or social worker can advise on how to tell children, for example, that their father is dying, or even explain it themselves. They will know what reassurance children are going to need, about what their father will look like, about death itself and about its causes — many young children may imagine themselves in some way responsible for the death.

It may also be necessary to dispel the fears of adults about the effect that seeing someone near death will have on a child. It is likely to be a well-meaning mistake to try to protect the child. The last moments that children and their parent or grandparent spend together may be very meaningful to both of them. Hospice staff will know what to advise for the best.

Families are highly complex. It is not easy at the best of times to fathom out why a son is behaving in a certain way, nor why a husband or wife is suddenly so hostile or bitter. With the impending death of someone much loved, it can be even harder to understand what is motivating another's actions, and to cope with them.

One man in a hospice was deeply hurt by the fact that his 16-year-old only daughter, to whom he had been very close, would rarely come to see him. He and his wife had not been able to acknowledge to each other the fact of his impending death, and both had made the daughter's behaviour the focus of their anxiety. Both accused her of not being any support to her mother. It was only the intervention of the social worker that enabled the daughter to reveal her fear, not just of losing her beloved father, but of being seen after his death as a crutch to her mother, and never being free to leave and live her own life.

In a family meeting, the mother was able to face up to her own unwillingness to confront the reality of her husband's death and what it would mean to her. In facing it and sharing her feelings, she was able to find her strength. Her husband became more cheerful and relaxed, and the daughter was able to express her own feelings for him without fear that she would be smothered by the need of either her father or her mother.

~

ALLEVIATING GUILT

Another very important role for professional staff is to reassure families that they need feel no guilt because they could no longer cope at home. Very often people think that they have failed if they cannot make the loved one comfortable and pain-free at home; or if, at a time when they expected to be most caring and giving, they find themselves feeling increasingly irritable and anxious.

A hospice admission is never seen as a family failure. It may be necessary on physical grounds or, just as vitally, to give the family an absolutely essential break. Very often strains that became so overwhelming at home disappear within days when the patient is settled and feels safe. Suddenly the pressure is off. There is the space for everyone to meet each other again, with much of the underlying anxiety and tension removed.

Conversely, there may be others who feel that their parent or spouse would be better off in professional hands and, effectively, bow out from playing any part in their care. It is a reaction often induced by fear. Staff can help the relatives to see that, even while the patient is in the hospice, there is much that the relatives themselves can contribute that will bring pleasure to them both. Relatives, as mentioned before, are never made to feel like intruders or amateurs in the care of the dying.

THE WAY OF DEATH

In our hearts, we all want a "good death" for someone we love. If we are aware of the hospice philosophy of care for the dying, we may feel even more acutely what we think it should be possible to achieve, in terms of communication and sharing, in the time a loved one has left. It can then come as even more of a shock, as my sister and I discovered, if things do not work out in the way we have visualised and wanted.

Hospice workers I spoke to all made a point of stressing that people choose their own way to die. Not everyone does acknowledge in any very obvious way the fact that they know they are dying, but that doesn't mean that, in their own way, they have not prepared for and accepted death. Some may say everything they want to say in a last squeeze of the hand. Some may say nothing at all.

Such a way of death may be harder for the relative than for the patient to accept. It is even hard for those who work in hospices and is a lesson that often has to be learned very early. As one hospice sister said: "We cannot have preconceived ideas about how we would like patients to die. Some do not accept death and a nurse may feel that, because the patient never opened up or talked at all, she must have failed him. But you can't force people into dying at peace, in your own terms, spiritually and emotionally. All we can do is offer all we have to give, for all who want it."

Family and friends, too, can aim for no more than that.

10.

HOME CARE, HOSPICE-STYLE

One of the most interesting developments within the hospice movement in recent years has been the spread of home care support services. They are enabling a great many more people to live out the last of their days in their own homes, with those they love and surrounded by all the things that are dear and familiar.

~

THE CONFIDENCE TO COPE

Hospice-style support for families at home is an important progression; the knowledge that it is available has given innumerable relatives the confidence to cope. How often have we all heard someone say: "I would so much have liked to care for her at home, but I thought she would be better looked after by professional people."

It is a very understandable fear. We may be frightened that we will not be good enough at making someone we love feel comfortable, that they may suffer pain which we won't be able to relieve, or that some crisis may suddenly occur with which we won't know how to cope. It feels like an awesome responsibility to be caring for someone who we know is going to deteriorate instead of getting better. Will we be able to deal with our own emotions, as we see that happen? Will it not, perhaps, be too painful to bear for absolutely everyone concerned?

Some people fear that, once the patient has come home and the hospital bed is quickly allocated to someone else, they will be left to cope alone without any support at all. Many general practitioners are very understanding and supportive indeed, but others may themselves be uncomfortable with the emotional aspects of death, and not have much to offer personally. To be assured that "it will be all right" or "you are doing your best" is not necessarily enough for the anguished relatives.

There is the quite justified fear that caring will be a 24-hour job, physically and emotionally exhausting. Would it not be worse to become so overtired and irritable that we end up snapping at the person we so much want to do our best by and making them feel a burden, rather than letting them stay in hospital with professional carers?

Sometimes, of course, families are confused and hurt when patients seem to rage at them and blame them for all manner of unexpected things, when they are trying hard to do their best. They do not understand that this is just a phase in the patients' own acceptance of their condition. They think, perhaps, that patients would *prefer* to be in hospital.

They may worry, too, that they will need so much in the way of aids and special equipment, of the type that they see in hospitals, that they will soon get out of their depth. Or they may be anxious about correctly administering the different doses of drugs.

These are the kinds of concerns that can quickly be overcome with the help and understanding of a home care team. About half of all hospices now have home care teams, so families who are given their services also have the comforting knowledge that the hospice is there in the background to provide a respite of in-patient care for the patient, should that ever become necessary or appropriate.

HOME CARE NURSES

There is also, however, a large and ever-growing number of home care nurses who are based in National Health Service health centres or hospitals, as well as in hospices.

The majority of these are Macmillan nurses. For the first two or three years, their salaries are paid by the National Society for Cancer Relief, founded by Douglas Macmillan, and are then taken over by the local health authority.

There are always at least two Macmillan nurses based in any one community, and very many districts try to have three or four. The nurses have usually worked as district nurses or health visitors before being specially trained to work with the dying.

ACCESS TO HOME CARE TEAMS

Sixty per cent of health districts now have access to specialist home care teams, either of their own or from a voluntary hospice. The National Society is working very hard to encourage the remainder to make special provision for dying patients; and, since December 1985, when the National Association of Health Authorities held a conference on terminal care, there has been a considerable increase in interest.

In 1984, there were a total of 260 Macmillan nurses in the community, who were able to help over 18,000 patients. There are, at the time of writing, now over 300 specially trained nurses, with a corresponding increase in the numbers of patients and families they can support. Home care, then, is a very realistic option for a great many families who want it.

~

ROLE OF THE HOME CARE TEAM

The home care team may consist of a single nurse or, in the case of the larger hospices, a group of professionals including a doctor and a social worker. Whatever the set-up, the home care staff are there to *advise* families, not to provide nursing care or to take over from anyone else. The home care teams work closely with a patient's general practitioner and with the district nurses. They do not interfere with each other's roles.

Just as all hospices differ in exactly how they perform their functions, so home care teams may have individual ways of working. I shall, however, use as an example the home care team at St Christopher's, which was established as far back as 1969, and from which many other hospices have drawn and developed their ideas.

At St Christopher's, there are five home care nurses, one of whom will always be on call at any hour of the day or night. They cover almost all of South-East London, a very densely populated area that is split among six health authorities.

REFERRALS

Patients are first referred to the home care team either by the doctor they have been under at the hospital, or by their own general practitioner. The general practitioner must fill in a brief medical form, explaining what the patients are suffering from, what operations or other treatments they have had, what drugs they are now taking, and what they know about their own condition.

Relatives are also asked to fill in a form, saying why they would like assistance from the home care team.

THE FIRST VISIT

All the requests received are reviewed at a daily meeting at the hospice. Families whom it is felt would immediately benefit from help very quickly receive a 'phone call from a member of the home care team to arrange a visit. Or the visit may be to a person with cancer who is living alone.

Sometimes relatives ask the home care team to pretend that they have come from somewhere other than a hospice — frightened that, if they don't, the patient will then realise that they must be dying. This is not a request that the team can grant. To be dishonest at the start would make it very hard later, and justly so, for the team to gain the patient's trust.

The first visit always takes place within a week of when the application is received. And families are warned that it is likely to be a long visit (one to two hours) because there is a lot of ground to cover.

At St Christopher's, the first visit is made by a nurse. (In some other home care teams, it is the doctor who makes the initial contact.) The first thing the nurse does is to take down a very detailed history. Patients are asked everything, right from the start, from what symptoms they first had and when they first realised something was wrong, through their hospital treatment, to how they feel now. How is their appetite? Are they constipated? Do they have any swelling, or any difficulty in breathing? Do they have any problems in getting about, or in moving any particular part of the body?

The nurse will want an extremely clear picture of the degree of pain patients are suffering, for symptom control is the very first priority, just as in in-patient care. Patients will be asked if the pain is a dull ache or the stabbing kind, if it is continuous or intermittent, and how long any drugs the doctor may have prescribed stay effective.

The nurse will also gently assess how much the patients — and their families — actually know about their condition. Even if the general practitioner has indicated on the original application form that everyone knows everything, the nurse will not in fact assume that this is the case. As mentioned previously, patients sometimes choose to "forget", and relatives are sometimes presumed to have understood more than they really have. For instance, an embarrassed consultant may have talked in technical terms, leaving the relatives confused and uncertain about what the patient's future hopes really are.

The final important thing to find out, on this first visit, is the circumstances of the family members themselves. Are there a number of people available to share the care, and offer each other support? How well does everyone get on with one another? If there are strains between the patient's husband and sister, for example, and differences of opinion about how she should be looked after, these may need to be tackled to prevent any problems from escalating as stresses increase. Is the person who is to be the main carer actually going to be available all the time, or will he or she need assistance? Are there children in the house whose needs must also be met?

ASSESSING NEEDS

Armed with as much information as possible, the nurse
will then meet with the other members of the home care
team at the hospice. These will include the other nurses,
two doctors and a social worker. Together they decide on
the best course of action.

They will determine what medication is necessary for
the patient, to relieve pain and any other discomfort. At
St Christopher's it is the practice to provide any drugs
themselves in the first instance, and then leave repeats to
be prescribed by the general practitioner (with the
exception of morphine, for which they use their own usual
chemist). The family doctor is kept informed throughout
of everything that is prescribed, or any changes that are
made to drug regimens.

The team will also think about the emotional needs of
the family. If, for instance, the family insists that they
don't want the patient to be told the truth about his or her
condition, that is something they will initially respect.
After all, it is the family members who are the ones who
are taking on the main burden of caring.

But the social worker will see the family to try to help
them overcome their fears about being honest, especially if
the patient wants the truth. Nothing is forced on the
families, nor are any decisions made on their behalf. They
are helped to move at their own pace, as and when they are
ready for it.

～

ARRANGING LATER VISITS

Within a day or two of this initial visit, the home care
nurse will again go and see patients to start them on their
new treatments, and to discuss anything they or their

families want to talk about.

From then on the visits vary according to need. Usually, someone from the hospice will 'phone once a week and visit once a week. But if a patient is in trouble, someone will come every day if needs be. Conversely, if the patient seems stabilised and the family is coping, contact just once a fortnight might be sufficient.

The length of visits also varies according to need. On average, they will range between 30 minutes and an hour. The team can always be 'phoned at any time, of course, but, in practice, night call-outs are rare. Often it is sufficient to give advice over the phone about how to handle a troubling symptom, or to put people's minds at rest about what a certain reaction or development may mean. The skill and success of the team, in providing pain relief and generating confidence in the carers, is proved by the fact that hospice doctors are very rarely called to see home care patients at all!

~

SUPPORT FOR THE FAMILY

The home care team sees its main role, after symptom control, as being there to listen to and assuage fears, both of patients and their families.

Relatives who are worried about whether the pain will get bad and uncontrollable at the end, or whether patients will become confused or start to shout, are assured that, in most cases, death is peaceful, and are told how each new symptom can be controlled as it arises. It is comforting to realise that fits, convulsions and haemorrhages, leading to death, are very very rare when symptom control is good.

If a family is under strain because either the patient or the relatives or both are unwilling to level with each other about the patient's true condition, a social worker is always on hand to help them and support them through the consequences of "telling" and being told.

Social workers also have a valuable role to play in helping adult members of the family to inform and support their children through what is happening; or to tackle any emotional difficulties that have arisen, such as teenage children acting rebelliously or withdrawing from the family, because of the unexpressed fears and tension in the house.

For, whereas parents may think it best that their children do not "trouble" grandad or grandma too much, or think it wiser to let them think he or she is recovering, the children may not read the circumstances in the same way. They may imagine that their grandparent doesn't love them anymore, or they may be confused and frightened by an unhealthily hushed and reverent atmosphere in the house, or resent the fact that they are not getting their due share of attention — and then suffer terrible guilt when their grandparent dies, thinking it was their fault. It is very often easier if someone skilled and sympathetic from outside the family can help parents broach these very difficult problems and offer reassurance and continuing support.

There may well, of course, be family crises to cope with which have nothing at all to do with the illness. These will inevitably add more strain to an already strained house, and social work support may be very helpful.

The social worker can also help the family in very practical ways, such as applying for grants for necessary aids or for meeting added expenses, such as heating. (See Chapter 12 for full details about grants.)

There is another honorary member of the home care team who has something very significant to offer: the volunteer. It can be a godsend indeed to have someone who is willing to collect children from school or do the Saturday shopping, to come and sit with the patient in the evening now and then, so the family can have a break, or, simply, to be there to chat to whoever feels like talking. Volunteers are well-trained and often become very experienced supporters, and their help is, of course, particularly valuable for a patient who lives alone.

As in the hospice in-patient units themselves (and, by the nature of the circumstances, perhaps even more so), members of the home care team are always ready to do bits of each other's jobs. The social worker will not say that it isn't for her to help make patients more comfortable in bed or walk them to the toilet. The nurse will be just as ready to talk with the members of the family about their fears as concern herself with the practical needs of the patient.

One of the home care nurses at St Christopher's said: "For all of us, our work is very much the sharing with the family of the pain and distress of seeing a loved one dying. We have found that families appreciate that very much. Just being there and sharing is often, in itself, enough."

GETTING A BREAK

Caring for a terminally ill relative at home is undoubtedly a 24-hour a day business. If patients are unable to get out and about easily, or at all, it can become very wearing for them, and for their main carers, to have to spend so much time cooped up in the same place.

Visits to an out-patient's clinic or to a day centre, where these are available, may do much to relieve boredom and tension, as well as having other physical and psychological benefits for patients. For the relatives, such visits can mean a well-earned rest or, if they choose to go along too, a chance for a reassuring or informative chat with relevant members of a hospice staff.

OUT-PATIENT CLINICS

A number of hospices run their own out-patient clinics. Usually, volunteers with cars are available to drive those who have no transport or who live alone to their appointment. Despite the fact that the meeting is medical rather than social in intent, very many people look forward immensely to their trip.

In purpose-built hospices, the out-patient clinic will be a very attractive and informal place, with comfortable easy chairs and plants, and pleasant paintings to look at in the waiting area.

There is plenty of time to talk with and ask questions of the hospice doctors who are running the clinic. And an opportunity can easily be made, if necessary, for relatives to see the doctor alone, if they have concerns they want to share in private — something that may be difficult sometimes, according to individual circumstances, when the nurse is visiting at home.

DAY CENTRES

Even more eagerly anticipated by a great many patients is the visit to the day centre, again with the help of volunteer drivers. A number of the larger hospices have such a centre, where people who are being cared for at home or who live alone can come once, twice or sometimes three times a week.

More and more day centres are likely to become available in the near future, especially as the National Society for Cancer Relief is also directing funds towards the setting up of Macmillan day units within National Health Service hospitals.

The day centre has several functions. It gives the

patient a break from home and a chance to meet and talk with other people. Lunch and tea are provided, so it is quite a social occasion. There is also an opportunity for doctors to pop in informally and see how people are getting on. Patients will meet others who work in the in-patient unit too, and thus become familiar with the hospice and its staff. This is an advantage for them if, at any later stage, they need admission themselves.

The mainstays of the day centre, however, are usually the physiotherapist and/or the occupational therapist. The physiotherapist can work there with patients to help them exercise their limbs, or to teach them how to adapt to any increasing disability so that they can keep their independence for as long as possible. The occupational therapist will also do everything possible to help people carry on managing for themselves at home, perhaps by showing them simple alternative ways to do something like manage a kettle or hold a cup.

The occupational therapist also arranges whatever work or leisure pursuits are on offer in the centre. These may include the opportunity to make simple crafts (the achievement of which can give a lot of pleasure), to paint, to grow flowers in window boxes, or simply to sit and knit and chat with neighbours. Those who enjoy being more actively social often enjoy a game of bingo or playing chess.

The day centre is a very good way to bridge the gap, when a patient could benefit from more than just an out-patient consultation with a doctor but doesn't need in-patient admission. Relatives are very grateful for the chance to relax alone, in the comforting knowledge that their loved one is in excellent care.

ADMISSION IF REQUIRED

When a home care team is backed by a hospice in-patient unit, there is always, of course, the reassuring knowledge that, if symptom control becomes impossible at home, or the strain of caring, perhaps because of other commitments and worries, becomes temporarily too much, the patient will always be able to have a hospice bed for as long and as often as necessary.

It may be the case that someone's symptoms only become too difficult to control at home very shortly before their death, and so in the event they die in the hospice rather than at home. This can be very upsetting to relatives who had so strongly wanted their loved ones to die where they had most liked to live, and they may feel a very painful sense of regret and failure. Yet, in reality, they will have done and given everything that they possibly could. If even the home care team believe at a certain point that someone will feel most safe and truly comfortable in the hospice itself, with all emergency aid on hand, the relatives can be reassured that hospice care, for those final days or hours, really must be what is best for everyone concerned.

But it is not the norm for admission to be necessary. And, according to members of home care teams, most relatives are very happy and very very glad that they were able to care for loved ones at home, sharing something very special and lasting together, which is what good memories are made of.

11.

SUPPORT IN BEREAVEMENT

When someone we love dies after an illness, it is for them the end of suffering; but for us it is only the beginning of a new kind of pain. The death of someone close, however much expected, however much prepared for or however much superficially it may seem a relief, is always when it actually happens much more of a shock than we had anticipated.

Hospice philosophy is not to say, "I'm sorry" when the inevitable end comes, and leave it at that. Hospices care for relatives as well as for patients, and they see it as their role to help people both to grieve and to cope with bereavement.

STAGES OF GRIEVING

Even if the loved one's death was indeed a relief because it signified an end of their suffering or sadness, the grief that follows is none the less for that. It has been suggested by experts that, when someone close dies, it takes at least two years fully to finish grieving, and often a great deal longer than that.

The depth of the emotions that people experience can be very scary, especially if they thought they were well-prepared and would manage to cope. First, there may be complete numbness or disbelief that the loved one has actually died. When that sinks in, the feeling of shock may give way to feelings of desperation and panic. Depending upon the relationship with the person who has just died, there may be feelings of not wanting to go on living without them, or of terrible loneliness and purposelessness; or, perhaps, there will be feelings of rage towards them for leaving us, or for getting ill in the first place. Certain feelings we have may seem inexplicable or unforgiveable to us, and we start to wonder if we are very heartless, or very selfish or worthless as human beings.

Very often, in our grief, we may start to experience worrying physical symptoms ourselves — an inability to sleep, loss of appetite, an irritable bowel. Sometimes we even feel we are experiencing exactly those symptoms which so upset us in the person who died, such as difficulty in breathing or an inability to swallow.

Very many people have such intense reactions. They may also feel obliged to put a brave face on the future, for the benefit of other people, or sense that others do not feel comfortable in the presence of such grief and so try to suppress it, for fear of being abandoned by them when they can lease bear to be alone.

But grief cannot successfully be suppressed. The feelings must go somewhere. Sometimes they may turn inwards, so that unexpressed guilt, that perhaps we could have done more or better by the loved one, festers into bitterness that pervades our whole outlook on life. Or the feelings manifest themselves as tension and take their toll on the body. People who are hard hit by bereavement, and who don't have adequate outlets or support, are at higher risk of mental or physical illness themselves.

ENCOURAGING GRIEF

For all these sorts of reasons, hospice staff believe that grief must be encouraged and supported. Many have their own bereavement counsellors who are there to help people who may, for a number of reasons, be at very serious risk. For those who do not need help to allow themselves to grieve, the acknowledgment from hospice staff of the depth of their loss and their feelings for the one who has died is in itself much appreciated.

Good hospice practice is to keep a record of individual family circumstances and their attitudes and reactions during the time when the loved one is dying, so that staff are quickly aware of who may be glad to receive help from bereavement counsellors when the time comes.

People are, for instance, much more likely to have difficulty in coming to terms with a death if the person who has died was the only one with whom they had a close relationship; or if they have only recently lost someone else, or perhaps have endured the deaths of several friends and relatives in a small number of years. If they had never fully acknowledged that the loved one was really dying, or are too self-blaming and reproachful after the death, they may not be able to cope with the intensity of their feelings.

It may be harder for a young mother who has to meet the demands of her children to allow herself due time to grieve for her own mother's death. If she is a single parent, the stress will be even greater.

Perhaps someone else in the household is sick, or there are marital problems which have just been "on hold" while attention was directed towards a parent or sister or brother of the spouse.

If other members of the family are not supportive and there are no close friends, grief may become suppressed. If, on the other hand, someone has suddenly a great deal of time on their hands, there may be little for them to do but dwell on their feelings. Someone who is unemployed, or retired and at home alone a great deal, will find it particularly hard to face the emptiness that follows a period of intense daily and demanding involvement with the dying person.

Justifiable worries about what will happen in the future will, naturally, make adjustment significantly worse — someone may be forced to move out of a house, for instance, or have no clear idea about how they will now support themselves financially. Pending upheavals of a practical nature, coupled with the huge emotional upheaval of loss, can precipitate physical illness or depression that may even lead to a suicide attempt.

These are just some of the kinds of family situations which hospice counsellors will want to be aware of. It is common practice for someone from the hospice who is familiar with the case, or a member of the home care team if the patient was cared for at home, to 'phone or visit the family a little while after the funeral.

Until the funeral is over, and all the practicalities of a death are out of the way, members of the bereaved family may often not give way to the fullness of their feelings. For there is much busying about to be done, much comfort, and condolences from relatives, friends and neighbours being offered in that time.

It is afterwards, when the yawning abyss in their lives is first fully apparent — and when the relatives and friends have often ceased to ring or call, embarrassed at not having anything they see as practical or useful to offer — that a visit from someone who cared for the patient and knew them as they were at the end is most to be appreciated.

It is at this time that, if it seems appropriate, further help from bereavement counsellors will be offered.

~

THE EXPRESSION OF GRIEF

Many of us feel uncomfortable about death and do not know how to behave when we are with a person who has just lost someone who was very close to them. Often it feels safer to try and keep their mind off the fact, and we make vain attempts to bring them out of themselves. Or we breezily ask, "How are you?" and hope that we will receive the brief answer "Fine", without any unloading of intense emotion that we fear we may not be able to handle. If we do this, it is out of embarrassment and uncertainty, and not from lack of caring.

But often it is only those who have been through the experience of bereavement themselves who know that something more needs to be offered. (Sometimes, however, someone who is still struggling to cope with a bereavement of their own finds it particularly hard to face someone else's grief.)

If the bereaved person does not have a close friend or family member who can fully support them in the pain and the slow readjustment to life without their loved one, a professional person or someone skilled in offering support has a great deal of value to offer. Hospices with bereavement support schemes train their staff and/or volunteers on how to encourage the expression of grief, and help people through it in a positive way. Not only will they visit for as long and as often as they are wanted, but they are also always at the end of a 'phone, if someone ever suddenly feels desperate and longs to talk.

According to a number of research projects examining bereavement services, the first benefit of this kind of visit is that bereaved people feel relief at being *allowed* to talk about the one who has died. They may want to go over what it felt like for them while the loved one was ill or at the moment of death, or else describe the funeral — matters about which, a fortnight after a death, well-meaning friends tend to discourage discussion because it seems to them unnecessarily morbid.

However, such intense feelings, and memories of such a painful time, do not disappear so rapidly. A woman who has just lost her husband or her mother may need to recount and relive the experience a number of times, before she can fully accept it and express all her sadness about it.

It is important to feel the sadness and not fight it or deny it. Otherwise it will stay inside somewhere, suppressed but not subdued, and ready to burst forth at a much later and, perhaps, unexpected time.

Bereavement counsellors (a term I am only using for simplicity, as the person offering support could be a nurse, a social worker, a chaplain or a volunteer) can offer tremendous reassurance just by showing in their responses that intense grief is natural, and by accepting whatever the bereaved person wants to express. Relatives often say things like, "You are the first person who has really understood what it was like". This is not a poor reflection on family and friends, but an acknowledgment of the fact that grief can sometimes be hardest to share with those close to us, who also have their own memories and sadness or remorse.

It helps too, to learn from someone "outside" that to feel anger or guilt is very common, and is not a sign of cracking up or of being an unworthy person. Again, these feelings will be encouraged, even if they are uncomfortable to handle (anger may be directed towards the counsellor, for instance, until the bereaved reach a point where they realise the anger is in fact for themselves, at being left perhaps, or at being unable to have done more for the dying person).

The counsellor will not criticise, but when appropriate

will do more than just listen. It is of no lasting help to let anger or guilt slide into bitterness. That can last for years, and spill over into all of a person's life. When the moment is right, the counsellor will therefore try to encourage acceptance instead of self-reproach, and help sow the seeds of new hope.

SUPPORT FOR CHILDREN

Help may also be needed where children are concerned. When we are feeling so disoriented and desperate ourselves, it can be difficult to allow ourselves to accept that young children may be suffering in the same way as well. We don't want them to suffer, just as friends and family want us to stop suffering, but wanting does not make their pain any less profound.

Counsellors can be a pillar of strength when people have to try and cope with the grief of others in the family as well as their own.

PRACTICAL PROBLEMS

During this period, there may be practical problems which a professional can very much help with — sorting out finances, arranging things around the house, ensuring that the children are taken care of.

The counsellor will no doubt know of all the local and national organisations that can help with particular problems, and also of any voluntary self-help groups which may have something special to offer.

MOVING NATURALLY THROUGH SORROW

Experts believe it is better to stay with the grief for as long
as is necessary, to move through from the stage of disbelief
and the feeling that life has no more meaning for us, to the
point where we can get back in touch with our good
feelings about the lost person's life, the value it had for us
and for them, and the realisation that what we shared is a
treasure that can never be taken from us — indeed, that
what we learned from that person, and enjoyed and
remember, is something we ourselves take on into the
future.

For that reason, hospice philosophy is not to dampen
down initial pain with tranquillisers or anti-depressants,
so that we cease to be in touch with it and are unable to
work with it. Deep sorrow is natural. Nor is it "best" to
put away all photos of happier times that act as sad
reminders, or to attempt to escape from the sense of the
dead person's presence by rushing to move house and
take a job in a completely different area. These are
attempts to suppress grief, but they may cause more
despair and loneliness, rather than less.

AN END TO GRIEVING

As Dr Colin Murray Parkes has put it, the time will
eventually come, if the sorrow is allowed to take its
natural course, when a person may need "permission" to
stop grieving. Here again, the support of an experienced
and sympathetic outsider can be so important. For, when
the grief starts to lessen, sometimes we can feel guilty at
finding ourselves wanting to take an interest in life again,
and open ourselves to new experiences and perhaps new
people.

It may feel disloyal to the husband or wife who has died, or to the much-loved sister. How can we allow ourselves to feel happy or positive and energised when they are no longer with us? Yet those who have had experience of death and bereavement know that grief that is expressed eventually runs its course, and that though the feelings for the person who has died will never disappear, we still have our own life force to which, eventually, we will want to respond in whatever way is right for us.

Hospice philosophy is that not only is death itself a natural part of life, but so is bereavement. By facing both, instead of fearing them, and by trusting our own feelings, we can survive the pain and carry on with a much deeper and more connected sense of life itself. Hospices are themselves evidence of that. No one could work in a hospice and have so much to give to others suffering emotional and physical pain, if he or she did not believe in life.

~

THE FOLLOW-UP

It means a lot to relatives to know that the loved ones who died were also important to the people who nursed them as professional carers. Hospice staff who became particularly close to a patient may want to attend the funeral, although that is not always possible. It is certainly common for a periodic telephone call to be made to the nearest relative, whether or not they need bereavement support, just to see how they are getting on. A card may be sent on the first anniversary of the death, to say that hospice staff are thinking of the bereaved. There may be a memorial service arranged at the hospice.

SUPPORT GROUPS

Many bereaved relatives have derived significant support from attending an evening group once a month, arranged through various hospices, at which they can share their feelings with others who have also known grief. Some may come only a few times; for others, particularly the elderly living alone, it may be a welcome lifeline.

Studies have compared what happened to people after a loved one died in hospital and no help was offered in bereavement, and what happened to those who had the benefit of hospice-style care and counselling. The results show clearly the benefits of a bereavement support scheme. Relatives who received support were far less likely, nearly two years later, to suffer from anxiety and physical ill-health, or to rely for support on drink, tranquillisers and smoking.

Relatives who had known that the patient was going to die, and who were helped to "grieve" before as well as after, later experienced a much greater peace of mind. They also had far fewer distressing memories when the patient had not died in unrelieved pain and they had not felt powerless to help — strong testimonials indeed to the whole hospice philosophy of care.

12.

HOW TO FIND HELP

AVAILABILITY OF HOSPICE-STYLE CARE

Hospice-style care is now available in a great many parts
of Britain and Eire, although, unfortunately, not all. At
the beginning of 1986, there were over 90 in-patient units
(providing, in all, over 2,000 beds) and over 120 home care
or hospital support teams. There were also another 40 new
hospice projects, both in-patient and home care, in the
pipeline for completion by the end of 1987.

Their geographical spread is very wide and spans most
counties. However, hospices usually operate on a
catchment area system; that is, they take patients only
from a specific locality around them. Exceptions can be
made in some very special circumstances, so it is always
worth finding out, even if you are unlucky enough to live

in an area that is not served by hospice-style facilities.
But hospices are not normally happy to take patients
whose relatives are going to have to travel a long way in
order to see them.

~⚬~

FINDING A HOSPICE

Your own general practitioner should know whether there
is a hospice or home care team in your particular area. If,
however, you wish to do some finding out for yourself and
do not want to ask your doctor in the first instance, you
can ring the Hospice Information Service (address and
telephone number on page 120) or send a large stamped
addressed envelope to receive their directory of hospice
services. They keep an up-to-date list of all hospices and
home care services, and of all hospitals which have special
wards or teams of specialist advisory staff (known as
symptom control teams).

You can then, if you like, ring the hospice which is in
your area to find out more about how it works or what it
offers. In most cases the care is free, but a very few have
to make charges.

~⚬~

APPLYING FOR A PLACE

The application has to come from the patient's own
general practitioner, or hospital doctor. You cannot apply
by yourself.

Occasionally, some general practitioners do not like the
idea of involving a hospice. They may feel that they
themselves know the patient best, and resent what they

see as an intrusion on their own patch. Hospices in fact always fully involve the general practitioner, but there may still be some who are resistant in principle.

Unfortunately, in such a case, there is no way to get round the fact that you need the doctor's permission. You may have to be very persistent or, perhaps, even insistent. One hospice doctor said: "There are some families who have had to take the application form to the general practitioner, lie on the floor and kick and scream until he filled it in." But the likelihood of meeting such hostility is rare, as general practitioners become more aware of what hospices can offer, and more keen to work alongside hospice staff.

It is a very good idea to make an application to a hospice early, perhaps shortly after a diagnosis of incurable cancer, and well before the time when the patient may need the bed. All sorts of delays can occur, when forms have to be filled in and sent by post, and hospice staff also like a little time, unless admission is urgent, to acquire all the information they can about the patient and the family they are going to help. Matters can be handled more smoothly and much more speedily if a hospice already "knows" about a prospective patient, and is ready to act quickly when the time comes.

WAITING LISTS

Hospices do have waiting lists, however. Some prefer to call them priority lists, as they will endeavour to give help first to whoever has most need, physical, emotional or spiritual. It will be the hospice's own decision when and if they can help you. Most, for instance, only take people who are suffering from incurable cancer, although about a third have one or two beds for sufferers from motor neurone disease.

Patients do not have to be of a particular religion, or indeed to have any religion at all.

~~

THE RIGHT TIME

Your own doctor should be able to help you decide whether you might need hospice help, and at what stage. For instance, patients may benefit from a week's admission early on, to get their symptoms under control, and then be able to go back home again. They may not need to return to the hospice for months or even, in some cases, years — or perhaps not at all.

Others may benefit from day care or out-patient facilities, but may not want in-patient hospice care till towards the end of their lives, when they may need on-the-spot, expert attention to deal with discomforts, or when the strain may have become too much for relatives.

~~

HOW LONG TO STAY?

Lengths of stay will vary according to individual circumstances. They may range from two days to several months. No one is "made" to stay longer than they wish nor to leave, if they can leave, before they are ready.

But hospices can offer most, with their special skills, if patients who are to die in in-patient units are with them for at least two weeks; otherwise there may not be enough time for staff and patients to get to know each other as personally as they would like, or to offer full emotional support.

PRE-ADMISSION CONTACT

Patients and/or relatives may well be offered the chance to come and look around the hospice beforehand, and to chat with staff about any worries. Similarly, hospices generally like to have made contact with a family themselves before a person is admitted.

In some cases, it may be the hospice doctor who visits a patient at home or in hospital. In others, it may be the home care sister or the social worker who comes to the patient's house. An initial visit like this is useful not only for the staff, who can start to assess needs, but for the patient who may have some basic worries (such as, "Will I be allowed to take my pipe?") which can quickly be sorted out.

~

FINDING HOME CARE HELP

If you are hoping to take care of a relative at home and feel that you would like more support than your general practitioner has time to offer, he or she will know whether there is a hospice with a home care team operating in your area, or whether there are home care nurses based at the local hospital or health centre. You can, however, enquire for yourself from the Hospice Information Service (page 120), or by contacting the National Society for Cancer Relief (page 121) to ask about Macmillan nurses.

Family doctors have to approve of their involvement, as they and the district nurses will be working very closely with them. Again, it is general practitioners who make the initial approach. The home care team will work in an advisory and supporting capacity only, while the general practitioner stays firmly in charge of the patient's overall care.

There are other organisations which may be able to help
if you are caring for someone at home. The Marie Curie
Memorial Foundation (page 121) can supply nurses and
night-sitters in certain areas, or there may be local
volunteers. Your district nurse or doctor will know
whom to contact.

GRANTS FOR HOME CARE

If you are caring for a patient at home, you may be eligible
to apply for certain grants. The National Society for
Cancer Relief (page 121) has a Patient Grants Department
to which applications are made for people in need by
health authority or hospice social workers. Every
application is considered as quickly as possible; and grant
money, when awarded, is sent out within a week or so of
when the application was received.

Examples of needs for which grants have been given
include home help, night or day nursing, fares for relatives
to visit, food, heating, bedding, holidays, and domestic
appliances.

SELF-HELP SUPPORT ORGANISATIONS

Whether your relative is being cared for in a hospital, a
hospice or at home, you may welcome being in touch with
other people who are currently facing the same sort of
anxieties.

There are a number of self-help organisations which
specialise in supporting people who have, or whose
relatives have, cancer; many also offer an information

service. Details of these appear below, along with the
addresses of organisations already mentioned, and others
which may be helpful to you.

~

USEFUL ADDRESSES

British Association of Cancer United Patients
(BACUP)
121-3 Charterhouse Street
London EC1M 6AA
Tel: 01-608 1785/6
(An information service contactable in office hours to help
cancer sufferers, and their friends and families, to
understand more about the illness, and to provide
practical advice on how to cope.)

CancerLink
46 Pentonville Road
London N1 9HF
Tel: 01-833 2451
(A support and information service for people with cancer
and their families. Instigates the formation of support
groups, and can provide a directory of all existing support
groups on request.)

Compassionate Friends
5 Lower Clifton Hill
Clifton
Bristol
Avon
Tel: 0272 292778
(Can put bereaved parents in touch with self-help groups
and counsellors.)

CRUSE
Cruse House
126 Sheen Road
Richmond, Surrey TW9 1UR
(Local branches can offer support and advice to widows,
widowers and their children.)

Friends of Shanti Nilaya
Old Cherry Orchard
Forest Row
East Sussex
(Shanti Nilaya is Sanskrit for "home of peace", and is the
name of the centre established by Dr Elisabeth Kubler
Ross in California, where she holds workshops for people
who are dying or bereaved in order to help them come to
terms with grief. Friends of Shanti Nilaya carries out
similar support work in England.)

Help the Hospices
BMA House
Tavistock Square
London WC1H 9JP
Tel: 01-388 7807
(Acts as a national voice for the hospice movement and
raises funds at a national level, mainly for training and
education, to spread hospice expertise. Also grants money
for hospice projects.)

Hospice Information Service
St Christopher's Hospice
Lawrie Park Road
London SE26 6DZ
Tel: 01-778 1240/9252
(Provides information about hospice-style care available
in Britain and Eire. A full directory is available on receipt
of a large s.a.e.)

National Society for Cancer Relief
15-19 Britten Street
London SW3 3TY
Tel: 01-351 7811
(Provides financial assistance for patients and relatives in
need through its Patient Grants Department. Applications
should be made by local authority, hospital or hospice
social workers. The society also funds home care
[Macmillan] nurses in the community and in National
Health Service hospitals.)

The Marie Curie Memorial Foundation
28 Belgrave Square
London SW1X 8OQ
Tel: 01-235 3325
(A national charity which runs homes providing care for
the dying, and which offers nursing services for the dying
in local communities.)

Sue Ryder Foundation
Sue Ryder Home
Cavendish
Suffolk CO10 8AY
Tel: 09787 280252
(A national charity which runs a number of homes,
including several for people with advanced cancer.)

ABOUT THE AUTHOR

DENISE WINN is a freelance writer and journalist specialising in medical and psychological topics.

A former editor of *Psychology Today* and of the magazine produced by MIND (National Association for Mental Health) she is the medical writer for *Cosmopolitan* and contributes regularly to other magazines and newspapers.

She has written seven books. *Below the Belt — A Woman's Guide to Genito-Urinary Infections,* is also published by Optima.

In writing *The Hospice Way* Denise Winn brings insight from her own personal experience: she and her sister nursed their mother while she was dying of cancer.

More books from Optima ...

FRIENDS OF THE EARTH HANDBOOK
edited by Jonathon Porritt
A great many people are interested in protecting the
environment, but are not sure what they should do about it.
This is a practical guide on how to put environmental ideals into
practice.
   Topics discussed include the best ways to save energy, waste
disposal, the use of water, transport policies, the protection of
wildlife and the politics of food.
ISBN 0 356 12560 2
Price (in UK only) **£4.95**

YOUR BRILLIANT CAREER by Audrey Slaughter
This handbook by Audrey Slaughter, well-known Fleet Street
editor, offers a wealth of very practical advice for women of all
ages on how to turn a job into a career, with information about
training and specific management skills, as well as self-
confidence and mental attitude.
   The book includes useful hints from women at the top, and
will be of real help to all working women.
ISBN 0 356 12705 2
Price (in UK only) **£4.95**

STONE AGE DIET by Leon Chaitow
Leon Chaitow, well-known nutritionist and author, explores the
idea that the diet of our Stone Age ancestors was not only
healthy, enabling them to develop the most stable society known
in world history, but also very much in keeping with modern
nutritional advice.
   The book is firmly based on the latest scientific research, and
includes a number of appropriate recipes.
ISBN 0 356 12328 6
Price (in UK only) **£4.95**

SELF HELP WITH PMS by Dr Michelle Harrison
One of the most comprehensive books available on the subject of
PMS (premenstrual syndrome), it covers *all* its symptoms, both
physical and mental, including the much publicised topic of
premenstrual tension. The forms of treatment are fully
described in clear, everyday language. Case histories and up-to-
date details of new research into treatment are also included.
  Illustrated with humorous but sympathetic line drawings,
this book is an indispensable guide for the large number of
women who suffer from this syndrome every month.
ISBN 0 356 12559 9
Price (in UK only) **£5.95**

MENOPAUSE THE NATURAL WAY
by Dr Sadja Greenwood
A comprehensive book that answers all the questions a woman
could possibly ask about the menopause. Myths about the
menopause are corrected and all medical details are clearly
explained in language that anyone can understand. All forms of
treatment for the problems associated with the menopause are
discussed, including the most up-to-date and controversial.
Includes case histories and is illustrated with humorous but
sympathetic line drawings, that complement the positive
approach of the book.
  It will be welcomed by every woman (and a lot of men) as a
complete, practical guide to promoting good health and avoiding
illness in the second half of life.
ISBN 0 356 12561 0
Price (in UK only) **£5.95**

ALTERNATIVE HEALTH SERIES
This series is designed to provide factual information and
practical advice about alternative therapies. While including
essential details of theory and history, the books concentrate on
what patients can expect during treatment, how they should
prepare for it, what questions will be asked and why, what form
the treatment will take, what it will 'feel' like and how soon they
can expect to respond.

1. ACUPUNCTURE by Michael Nightingale
Acupuncture is a traditional Chinese therapy which usually (but
not always) uses needles to stimulate the body's own energy and
so bring healing.
ISBN 0 356 12426 6
Price (in UK only) **£3.95**

2. OSTEOPATHY by Stephen Sandler

Osteopathy started in the USA in the 1870s, and has since spread to many other countries. It is a manipulative therapy, where the osteopath heals by adjusting the position of bones and tissues.

ISBN 0 356 12428 2
Price (in UK only) **£3.95**

BELOW THE BELT — A WOMAN'S GUIDE TO GENITO-URINARY INFECTIONS by Denise Winn

A simple factual guide to all the sexually transmitted diseases and vaginal infections women risk catching.

It covers all the long recognized diseases, such as gonorrhoea and syphilis, and the most up-to-date facts about all the new hazards — herpes, genital warts, chlamydia and AIDS.

Causes, symptoms in both yourself and your partner, and advice on treatment (including self-help) are clearly explained, as are the possible consequences of not seeking treatment.

A frank and direct account, firmly based on the latest medical knowledge.

ISBN 0 356 12740 0
Price (in UK only) **£3.95**

DOWN TO EARTH — A CALENDAR FOR THE RELUCTANT GARDENER
by Mike Gilliam with Alan Titchmarsh

DOWN TO EARTH, like the associated radio programme, is for every gardener who only wants to potter for a couple of hours at the weekend, and still expects results. There's one main, illustrated task for each week, plus topical tips on smaller 'odd jobs'. The style is lively, the approach not always orthodox, and subjects range widely — lawns, hedges, flowers, ponds, trees, even discouraging unwelcome cats. The emphasis is on the easy, instant results and maximum effect for minimum cost and effort.

ISBN 0 356 12704 4
Price (in UK only) **£4.95**

All Optima books are available at your bookshop or newsagent, or can be ordered from the following address:

Optima, Cash Sales Department,
P.O. Box 11, Falmouth, Cornwall.

Please send cheque or postal order (no currency), and allow 55p for postage and packing for the first book plus 22 for the second book and 14p for each additional book ordered up to a maximum charge of £1.75 in U.K.

Customers in Eire and B.F.P.O. please allow 55p for the first book, 22p for the second book plus 14p per copy for the next 7 books, thereafter 8p per book.

Overseas customers please allow £1 for postage and packing for the first book and 25p per copy for each additional book.

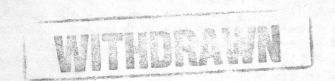